Endometriosis

CURRENT REVIEWS IN OBSTETRICS AND GYNAECOLOGY

OBSTETRICS

Series Editor

Tom Lind MB BS DSc PhD MRCPath MRCOG
MRC Human Reproduction Group, Princess Mary Maternity Hospital, Newcastle upon Tyne

Volumes published

Obstetric Analgesia and Anaesthesia 2E *J. Selwyn Crawford*
Early Diagnosis of Fetal Defects *D. J. H. Brock*
Early Teenage Pregnancy *J. K. Russell*
Drug Prescribing in Pregnancy *B. Krauer, F. Krauer and F. Hytten*
Aspects of Care in Labour *J. M. Beazley and M. O. Lobb*
Spontaneous Abortion *H. J. Huisjes*
Coagulation Problems during Pregnancy *E. A. Letsky*

Volumes in preparation

Immunology of Pregnancy *P. M. Johnson and H. Fox*
Ultrasound in Obstetrics and Gynaecology *W. J. Garrett and P. S. Warren*
Diabetic Pregnancy *M. Brudenell, M. C. Doddridge and P. J. Watkins*

GYNAECOLOGY

Series Editors

Albert Singer DPhil PhD FRCOG
Whittington Hospital, London
Joe A. Jordan MD DObst FRCOG
Birmingham Maternity Hospital, Queen Elizabeth Medical Centre, Birmingham

Volumes published

Ovarian Malignancies *M. S. Piver*
Cancer of the Cervix *H. M. Shingleton and J. W. Orr*
Female Puberty and its Abnormalities *J. Dewhurst*
Infertility in the Male *A. M. Jequier*

Volumes in preparation

Urinary Incontinence *S. L. R. Stanton, L. Cardozo and P. Hilton*
Endocrine Aspects of Female Infertility *M. Hull*

Daniel T. O'Connor
MB, BS(QLD), FRCOG, FRACOG

Visiting Gynaecologist, Royal
Brisbane Hospital, and Visiting
Gynaecologist, Cancer
Detection Clinic, Royal Women's
Hospital, Brisbane

Endometriosis

Series Editors
ALBERT SINGER AND JOE JORDAN

Churchill Livingstone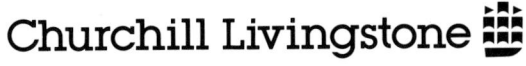

EDINBURGH LONDON MELBOURNE AND NEW YORK 1987

CHURCHILL LIVINGSTONE
Medical Division of Longman Group UK Limited

Distributed in the United States of America by Churchill
Livingstone Inc., 1560 Broadway, New York, N.Y. 10036, and
by associated companies, branches and representatives
throughout the world.

First published 1987

ISBN 0-443-02995-4
ISSN 0264-5610

British Library Cataloguing in Publication Data

O'Connor, Daniel T.
 Endometriosis.—(Current reviews in obstetrics and
 gynaecology, ISSN 0264-5610)
 1. Endometriosis
 I. Title   II. Series
 618.1′4   RG483.E53

Library of Congress Cataloging in Publication Data

O'Connor, Daniel T.
 Endometriosis.

 (Current reviews in obstetrics and gynaecology,
 ISSN 0264-5610)
 1. Endometriosis.   I. Title.   II. Series.
 [DNLM: 1. Endometriosis.   W1 CU8093M/WP 390 018e]
 RG483.E53025 1987   618.1′42   86-17153

Typeset by CCC, printed and bound in Great Britain by
William Clowes Limited, Beccles and London

Foreword

This series aims to present one person's overview of a clinical problem and in this book Dan O'Connor presents a unique assessment of the problem of endometriosis. He has reviewed, comprehensively, the world literature and based his conclusions on an exhaustive review of 717 cases of endometriosis personally diagnosed and managed. Many will be surprised that he demonstrated endometriosis, usually by laparoscopy, in one in 10 of all new patients seen by him between 1968 and 1983 and that one in 20 sufferers were teenagers. This latter group highlights his plea for early diagnosis by laparoscopy and that any management plan must consider the place of long-term suppression of menstruation as well as conservative surgery. The place of medical management of pseudopregnancy and pseudomenopause is described. No treatment is totally free of side-effects and the author's disillusionment with danazol (Danol) is obvious. However, the prospect of medical oophorectomy by the use of a gonadotrophin releasing hormone agonist and luteinising releasing hormone agonist offers an exciting new possibility.

For long the relationship between endometriosis and infertility has been known even when there seems to be no obvious reason why minimal areas of endometriosis should prevent pregnancy, but Dr O'Connor describes how recent work into the effect of endometriosis on the immune system may provide the answer.

In presenting such a large personal series of patients the author has given us a refreshing insight into a problem, often difficult to manage, which faces all gynaecologists and his conclusions are particularly relevant in that they are based on a combination of an extensive knowledge of published work and an obviously compassionate attitude to his patients: commendably he shows us how important it is that clinicians should never forget to treat the patient and not the disease!

London   Albert Singer
Birmingham   Joe Jordan
1987

Preface

Dramatic progress in most areas of obstetric and gynaecological practice has occurred in the last 20 years. Diverse topics have occupied centre stage during that time including, intermittently, endometriosis. Longstanding problems concerning this disease still, however, persist. It is still difficult to explain with confidence the aetiology of endometriosis to its sufferers because there is no simple explanation. It is likewise difficult to prevent the disease, and the many therapeutic programmes advocated in the past have always seemed to produce a hard core of failures and recurrences, a distressing and depressing situation for sufferers and those who care for them.

This book resulted from a visit to Brisbane in May 1981 by Joe Jordan. During his stay he attended one of my routine elective, non-selective gynaecological operating lists in St Andrew's Hospital and was intrigued by the number of cases of endometriosis, a number not thought to be unusual by the surgeon. He and Albert Singer subsequently asked me to write this book, suggesting that I tell about endometriosis as I understand it.

Many people have helped in the compilation of the manuscript. In particular, my wife, Liz, and family, uncomplainingly provided the time, space and support necessary to put it all together, my loyal friend and secretary, Marjorie Bierne SRN, and my daughter, Susan, typed the manuscript; my good friend Margaret Mason provided help with the graphic art work; longtime colleague and friend Dr Lawrence Brunello supplied a photograph of tubal endometriosis; and the Director General of Health, Dr P G Livingstone of the Queensland Government Department of Health, gave permission for the use of the brochure concerning hysterectomy. The publishers of *Contemporary Obstetrics and Gynaecology* gave permission for the use of a photograph illustrating Stage I endometriosis; Professor George Osbourne of the School of Veterinary Medicine at the University of Queensland advised on endometriosis in non-human primates; Mrs Elizabeth Drewe of the Australian Medical Association Queensland Branch Library kindly generated an extensive search of the literature; the enthusiastic and helpful staff of the Central Medical Library at the Royal Brisbane Hospital gave superb assistance; and Robert Hennig of Eldar Trading Company kindly provided the computer component.

Professor Robert Shaw of the Department of Obstetrics and Gynaecology in the Royal Free Hospital Medical School, London, most generously responded to a request from the publishers and kindly provided valuable information concerning a new medical approach in the management of endometriosis. He shared information obtained from his pioneering work concerning the use of gonadotrophin releasing hormone agonists in a series of patients with confirmed endometriosis that he has treated. This contribution has rounded out the text because I have had no personal experience with $GNRH_A$.

To all of the above a most heartfelt vote of thanks. The information in this book will, I hope, be useful not only in the educational situation but also when treating patients suffering from endometriosis. Meanwhile it is hoped that others will continue researching the many aspects of endometriosis that remain unclear so that the unanswered questions can be satisfactorily resolved for the benefit of patients with this vexatious disorder.

Brisbane 1987   D.O'C.

Contents

1. Introduction   1

    The Brisbane series   2
    Records and record analysis   4

2. Epidemiology   7

    Ethnic factors   7
    Age incidence   8
    Prior hormonal contraception   13
    Immunosuppressive drug therapy   13
    Hereditable factors   14
    Previous pelvic surgery   15
    Parity   15
    Coincidental disease   17
    Vaginal adenosis   18
    Genital tract epithelial dysplasia   19
    Incidence at exploratory surgery   19
    Endometriosis in the male   20
    Endometriosis in non-human primates   20

3. Aetiology and pathogenesis   24

    Ovarian morphology and function   26
    Immunological considerations   29
    Role of prostaglandins in endometriosis   32
    Hypothalamo-pituitary-ovarian axis factors   33
    Mechanical implantation factors   38
    Steroid receptors in endometriosis   39

4. Pathology and staging of endometriosis   44

    Gross pathology   44
    Endometriosis in other organ systems   50

Malignant tumours in endometriosis   54
Classification — staging of endometriosis   57

5. Clinical features and diagnosis   68

Symptoms   68
Signs   75
Diagnosis   78

6. Treatment of endometriosis   85

Surgical treatment   87
Results of surgical treatment   103
Medical treatment of endometriosis   112
Medical oophorectomy (based on a contribution by
   Professor Robert Shaw)   129

7. Hindsight   145

Index   149

1

Introduction

During a meeting of the Cambridge Medical Society on 14 April 1882, and reported in the *Lancet* of that year, Professor James Paget mentioned that many years before he had seen a young girl at Moorfields Hospital who, every month, had a small effusion of blood into the anterior chamber of her eye at the time of her menstrual period. This effusion was absorbed during the intervals between her periods.

Since this first record of the disease entity now known as endometriosis, interest and understanding of the disease have followed an erratic course with large gaps in our knowledge despite an increase in the volume of world literature.

This literature reflects many intriguing facets of this chameleon-like, ubiquitous disease process: the fact that there is no satisfactory single theory of aetiology; that this disease process affects not only human females and some males, but non-human primates as well; that no single therapeutic regimen suits all cases, and all stages of the disease, with equal expectations of success; that extended experience with conservative medical management seems so often to yield progressively less satisfactory results; and so on. One hundred years after the first somewhat offhand report of the disease entity, the omens suggest a much greater literature will need to accrue before the gaps in our knowledge of endometriosis are filled.

Twenty years ago, endometriosis was thought to be relatively uncommon, especially in public hospital patients, in Brisbane, Australia. While working in Guildford, England, during 1965 and 1966 the author was impressed by the fact that in Surrey at least, endometriosis was a relatively common disease amongst National Health Service patients and obviously there had to be other than geographic and ethnic factors operating to produce this disparity.

1

On returning to Brisbane in February 1967, Professor Eric Mackay of the Department of Obstetrics and Gynaecology, University of Queensland, introduced the author to the laparoscope and the first diagnostic laparoscopy was performed in that centre in March 1967. Undoubtedly this diagnostic procedure has led to an increased awareness of the possibility of endometriosis, diagnosis of the disease at an earlier stage in its natural history, and a subsequent apparent increase in its incidence. This has led to an increasing interest in the disease, and has resulted in increased referrals of potential endometriosis sufferers by aware, conscientious general practitioners who know of the author's special interest, so that a self-generating influence has occurred.

In keeping with the philosophy of this book a current review of the relevant international literature to April 1984 on the subject of endometriosis has been carried out. A review of a personal series of cases of endometriosis treated in Brisbane from February 1967 to January 1983, allowing a minimum of 12 months follow-up before compilation of data on these patients, will also be presented.

The Brisbane series

During the years analysed—February 1967 to January 1983—6656 patients were seen in consultation by the author in his private practice. During this time 760 cases of surgically diagnosed endometriosis were discovered of whom 717 were documented with sufficient accuracy to be included in an in depth survey. These 717 patients will be referred to throughout this book as the Brisbane series for ease of comprehension. Since I am not aware of any other Brisbane gynaecologist who has published a similar series I do not believe this to be an unduly arrogant or proprietary attitude, and use the description merely for convenience.

All the patients in the Brisbane series have been cared for in a private practice environment having been referred by general practitioners or other medical specialist colleagues. Undoubtedly 'word of mouth' referral from other patients initiated many consultations, and the author's known interest in this disease process has probably led to a biased incidence in referred patients.

During the years under consideration, private medical practice and a form of socialist public hospital medical care had coexisted in the state of Queensland, in Australia, for nearly two generations. Patients have easy access to a full range of medical, hospital, pharmaceutical, and diagnostic services in the public hospital system with no direct costs at the point of service. They are cared for, however, by a system, rather than by an individual as occurs in private practice, and the system includes medical and nursing undergraduates, postgraduate trainees, etc. During these years the medical, hospital, pharmaceutical and diagnostic costs of private patients were subsidized by voluntary private medical and hospital insurance schemes with a form of government subsidy covering some, but not all, of these services, with refunding of up to 85% of medical expenses. Private practice is entrepreneurial and competitive, and patients dissatisfied with the care, attention and results of treatment by individual gynaecologists can freely seek help elsewhere. About 50% of the population choose private medical care.

For 12 months during 1980–1981 the author was assisted by a postgraduate gynaecological trainee as part of an experiment to determine whether it was possible to train someone at a postgraduate level in a private practice milieu. This concept was accepted by the Royal College of Obstetricians and Gynaecologists and the experiment was, I believe, very successful. At no time did the trainee have sole unsupervised care of any of these patients but her interest and enthusiasm benefited all concerned. In all critical regards the patients in the series were under the sole and total care of the author.

Of the 717 patients in the Brisbane series 531 are classified as 'current attenders' having been seen in the last 2 years to January 1984. Sixty patients have not been seen during this time but have been traced at the general practitioner level, often in a distant part of the state of Queensland (for example 1200 miles away in the city of Cairns), or interstate. One hundred and twenty-six have been lost to follow-up and this group includes some 42 patients from such diverse places as Christmas Island in the Indian Ocean, the Kingdom of Tonga in the South Pacific Ocean, New Zealand, New Guinea, the Solomon Islands, Sweden and Vanuatu.

The population of Australia is polyglot with one-quarter born elsewhere, having voluntarily migrated to Australia in the last 30 years. Brisbane, a subtropical city with a population of one million (80 gynaecologists), services the state of Queensland which has a population of two million (a further 50 gynaecologists practising in non-metropolitan areas). It is also a port of entry for airlines from Papua New Guinea, New Caledonia, Vanuatu, the Solomon Islands, Fiji, New Zealand, Singapore, Hong Kong, Manila, and Tokyo as well as from the USA.

Aware that many of the traditional beliefs about endometriosis were liable to fall under close scrutiny in this current study, and having had the privilege of working in both the Kingdom of Tonga, and the Republic of Vanuatu (formerly the condominium of the New Hebrides), areas in the South Pacific populated by predominantly polynesian people and melanesian people respectively, the author knew that the belief that people from cultures regarded as unsophisticated by western standards rarely suffered from endometriosis, was just not true. Research into the countries of origin of the patients in the Brisbane series showed, not surprisingly (given the immigrant factor), that the 717 patients were born in Canada, Czechoslovakia, Denmark, Finland, France, Germany, Greece, Hungary, India, Indonesia, Iran, Ireland, Israel, Italy, Japan, Malaysia, Malta, Melanesia, Micronesia, The Netherlands, New Zealand, Norway, Poland, Polynesia, South Africa, Sri Lanka, Sweden, Switzerland, Thailand, UK, USA, Vietnam and Australia. It therefore seems reasonable to generalize that no ethnic group in this community seems particularly vulnerable, or immune, to endometriosis.

Records and record analysis

A very unsophisticated system of record keeping has been employed in the author's practice since its beginning and, prior to the invitation to write this book, there had been no pressing need to update the system. Colleagues at the medical school at the University of Queensland were consulted initially for help with information retrieval from patients' records and a system of retrieval using an unsophisticated method of data collection was organized and data painfully and tediously collected by systematically going through all patients' individual records, first to discover those surgically diagnosed as having endometriosis, and then to extract relevant information according to sets of relevant factors. Since, in the early years of the study, no attempt had been made to locate accurately or stage the disease, 43 patients' records were discarded as being inadequate for the survey. The medical school staff could not cope with the flood of information derived from the records reviewed, so after a frustrating delay and disappointment, help was obtained from a private company for data entry and analysis.

Robert Hennig of Eldar Trading Company, knew nothing about endometriosis at the start of this project and the author knew nothing about computers. Eventually they constructed a data bank system using the VACS data base on an ONYX 800 Z mini-computer. The work done was limited to the totalling and reporting utilities of the data base only as there was not enough time to carry out elegant statistical programming and analysis. The data base design consisted of a main record for each patient with an identifying code number so that anonymity was preserved, and all relevant personal data such as date of birth, marital status, parity, contraceptive history, past medical, surgical, gynaecological and family history, etc. were recorded. To these main records were hung sub-records covering such areas as diagnostic operations, medical treatment, etc., to which in turn were hung further sub-sub-records of such matters as operative complications, results of treatment, etc. The results are held on magnetic tape for re-use, re-evaluation and updating as needed.

Caught up in the promise of newfound success with synthetic hormone therapy in endometriosis, and with expectations of a new trend in the progression and management of this disease, in 1964 the author enthusiastically entitled his gynaecological commentary submitted in his book required for the MRCOG examination, 'The hormone treatment of endometriosis'. Since then there have been espoused a series of disappointing and disillusioning concepts relating to the aetiology and management of endometriosis, especially the non-surgical management. The concept of an induced 'pseudo-pregnancy' state with synthetic progestogens as found in the oral contraceptive preparations; the pseudomenopause treatment with danazol; the reports from China of the remarkable effects of gossypol acetate in the treatment of endometriosis and adenomyosis; the role of immunological factors in the aetiology of endometriosis and associated infertility; the significance of luteinized unruptured follicles; the role of prostaglandin levels in the peritoneal fluid in endometriosis; and now the new prospect of 'medical oophorectomy', have all paraded across the international literature, but none of these modalities has provided a total answer to endometriosis.

In addition to the introduction of laparoscopy into gynaecological surgery, undoubtedly the second most important factor in the conservative management of endometriosis has been the development of microsurgical principles and techniques. A further addition to microsurgery has been the very modern supplementary therapy using laser surgery.

Notwithstanding, there are still a number of recurring unanswered questions about endometriosis:

Why does endometriosis persist and even progress in some patients during pregnancy and lactational amenorrhoea?

Why do neither pregnancy nor the oral contraceptive pill seem to protect patients against developing endometriosis?

What are the immune factors involved in the spread of this destructive disease process in individual patients?

Why do some males on oestrogen therapy in the course of treatment for prostatic disease produce tissue histologically identical with endometriosis?

Why is it that endometriosis and polycystic ovary disease seem to be commonly coexistent in Brisbane patients?

Why do so many adolescent females develop very significant disease after relatively few menstrual cycles?

Have altered attitudes in women and their expectations of normal feminine function influenced the apparent increase in the incidence of endometriosis?

Is physician orientated awareness responsible for earlier diagnosis? Does infertility cause endometriosis or result from it?

Why, in the author's hands in Brisbane, does danazol seem to be little more than an expensive and disappointing disaster rather than an effective therapeutic aid?

Why does in vitro fertilization seem to be less successful for those who have suffered from and been treated for endometriosis, than for other infertility patients?

Perhaps by the end of this current review these questions and other puzzles may be answered.

2

Epidemiology

There are no complete epidemiological studies of endometriosis available but this review of the relevant literature, together with information retrieved from the Brisbane series, will add to the pool of epidemiological knowledge.

Ethnic factors

The diverse origins of the 717 patients in the Brisbane series have been previously mentioned. It has been suggested in the past that there should be a lower incidence of endometriosis in underdeveloped countries where prolonged lactation is maintained for both infant welfare and contraceptive purposes. The author's experience— gained from working for 5 years in two South Pacific nations, the Kingdom of Tonga and the Republic of Vanatu—suggests that this is not true and in these countries it is not at all uncommon to find high parity, a history of prolonged lactation, endometriosis, and fibroids or pelvic inflammatory disease coexisting in one patient. The introduction of diagnostic laparoscopy into all communities should certainly reveal a higher than anticipated incidence of endometriosis.

During a 3.5-year period in Nigeria, Ekwempu & Harrison (1979) found 27 negroid Nigerians with endometriosis, an incidence of 8.2%, but in their series the location of the disease was very different to that of the Brisbane experience, being rare in the pouch of Douglas and absent from the recto-vaginal septum. Chatman (1976) and Miyazawa (1976) have both written of a similar incidence of endometriosis in American black women and Japanese women respectively. It is possible that one reason why endometriosis has not been previously suspected in some groups is ethnic variability in female response to pain, menstrual and coital incapacity and infertility. The spread of feminism and enlightenment may lead, in formerly unsophisticated communities, to an increased recognition of the clinical clues that often lead to a surgical diagnosis.

Age incidence

Traditionally endometriosis is said to be a disease of the fourth decade of life and the Brisbane series shows that 83% of patients were diagnosed by the end of the fourth decade (Table 2.1).

Table 2.1 Age distribution and marital and coital status

Age (years)	Total number	Single	Virgo intacta
0–15	3	3	3
16–20	42	31	13
21–25	121	40	19
26–30	154	14	2
31–35	161	13	2
36–40	107	10	7
41–45	82	3	1
46–50	37	2	2
51–55	7	—	—
56–60	2	—	—
61–65	1	—	—
Total	717	116	49

The adolescent patient

Thirty-five patients in the Brisbane series were aged between 14 and 19 years inclusive and three have been lost to follow-up. All had diagnostic conservative surgery and postoperative medical therapy. Eighteen of the 35 had coincidental pathology (Table 2.2). Three of the seven girls with pelvic inflammatory disease had a history of appendicectomy combined with 'ovarian cystectomy'. This potentially dangerous procedure is commonly performed around puberty in females with non-specific right iliac fossa pain or pelvic pain, and is often performed by surgeons who do not acknowledge the important role of laparoscopy in establishing an accurate diagnosis in this age group before unnecessarily interfering surgically. Consequently unnecessary mutilation of the abdominal wall, needless

Table 2.2 Endometriosis and coincidental pathology

Endometriosis + polycystic ovary disease (PCOD)	9
Endometriosis + pelvic inflammatory disease (PID)	4
Endometriosis + PCOD + PID	1
Endometriosis + cervical intra-epithelial neoplasia (CIN iii)	1
Endometriosis + PCOD + PID + CIN ii	1
Endometriosis + PID + CIN iii	1
Endometriosis + Blackledge syndrome	1
Total	18

interference with harmless functional follicular ovarian cysts, the compromise of a previously clean pelvis by the removal of a normal appendix with the risk of infection, and the disastrous ultimate complication of avoidable infertility in the long term, are unfortunately well recognized sequelae to these operations in many instances. Jansen (1982) drew attention to these problems in Australia, where many laparotomies in this age group are commonly performed by non-specialists.

Only two patients in this small series had coexistent congenital anomalies, both had complete duplication of the genital tract but neither had urological abnormalities. This is in contrast with the experience of Schifrin et al (1973) who reported a series of 15 adolescent patients with endometriosis, six of whom had congenital urinary tract abnormalities. However, as in this latter series, one of the patients in the Brisbane series presented at 15 years of age, having had only nine periods, with an acute abdomen associated with a moderately large pelvic mass. She was virgo intacta and laparotomy revealed an intact imperforate hymen occluding one of her vaginae with haematocolpos, haematometra, haematosalpinx, and endometriotic destruction of the ipsilateral ovary with extensive stage II disease involving the rest of her pelvic viscera. Following oophorectomy and conservative surgery she remained symptom-free on continuous progestogen therapy until she moved away from Brisbane 3 years ago. The other girl has since had two caesarean sections and a subsequent sterilization procedure and is one of the patients who has had multiple recurrences after each pregnancy.

Chatman & Ward (1982) found that laparoscopically diagnosed endometriosis in black teenagers accounted for painful menstrual dysfunction in 28 of 43 girls while acquired dysmenorrhoea was the dominant symptom in 78%. In the Brisbane series pain, either associated with periods or with intercourse, was present in 30 of 35

9

adolescents. In the other patients the diagnosis was made on routine examination when nodules were detected in the pouch of Douglas at contraceptive consultation (2), at colposcopic examination for cervical intra-epithelial neoplasia (CIN) on cytology report (1), colposcopic assessment in a diethylstilboestrol-exposed girl (1), and for menstrual tenesmus and rectal bleeding (1).

The approach of Goldstein et al (1980) was similar to that of the Brisbane series, menstrual pain incapacitating to the point of interference with usual activities being the major indication for performing diagnostic laparoscopy. While vaginal examination is often difficult and unsatisfactory in this age group, rectal examination is more rewarding and tenderness with or without nodularity along the utero-sacral ligaments and in the pouch of Douglas and anterior fornix, is almost diagnostic of endometriosis in this age group.

The specific emotional needs of teenagers, their body image problems, difficulties with regard to self-esteem and self confidence, fears for their reproductive future, and coincidental parental and family conflicts, make it essential to explain patiently to these girls the real nature of the disease process and the procedures to be carried out. A genuine empathy for adolescents is essential in the management of their gynaecological problems and 'active listening' is a critical part of the consultation as well as the adoption of a non-authoritarian attitude.

In Brisbane, with its subtropical climate, most adolescent females spend a considerable part of the year clad in swimming costumes, with bared abdomens, so surgical procedures that leave minimal abdominal scarring are important if an ongoing rapport between patient and gynaecologist is to be established. Since continuing medical treatment, following initial surgery, is mandatory in the single adolescent group, and since adolescents are notoriously fickle in their adherence to any sort of regimentation including the regular routine taking of medication, it is particularly important that a mutual bond of trust and reliability be developed between gynaecologist and patient.

Because the opportunity to test reproductive potential may not occur for many years for these adolescents, and because the factors that led to endometriosis occurring in the first instance are probably still operative, it is likely that without ongoing post-surgical medical treatment recurrences will certainly occur.

Conflict often arises with the adolescent patient's parents over what is seen as meddlesome interference with normal biological activity, especially the induction of amenorrhoea, but a written explanation is usually sufficient to allay the fears of the parents in this matter. It is important at all times for the physician to consult the patient about her wishes in the area of family communication. In the Brisbane series the results 12 months after the initial diagnostic and therapeutic surgery and initial continuous progestogen therapy, which has been the basic modality used in this group, demonstrate a low cure rate (Table 2.3).

Table 2.3 Outcome in adolescent group within 12 months of primary surgery

Persistent symptoms	5
Persistent signs	6
Recurrent symptoms and signs	2
Cure	22
Total	35

One 17-year-old patient with coincidental polycystic ovary disease and persistent dysmenorrhoea, pelvic tenderness, and menstrual bladder dysfunction, was given a trial of danocrine, 200 mg twice daily after laparoscopic fulguration of multiple Stage I deposits scattered over her pelvic peritoneum and the surface of her left ovary, since neither continuous norethisterone, dydrogesterone, nor medroxyprogesterone controlled her problems. The use of danocrine proved disastrous as she experienced alarming virilizing effects and her voice was adversely affected with vocal cord hypertrophy persisting for 2 years after the cessation of therapy. This catastrophic complication to her career in the performing arts led to serious emotional distress and depression and needless to say this patient now regards all well-intentioned gynaecological advice with suspicion.

Since adolescents quickly tire of prolonged oral medication, 3-monthly injections of medroxyprogesterone acetate 150 mg/ml have proved most useful as a medical therapeutic agent in this age group, as will be discussed in greater detail in Chapter 6.

Postmenopausal patients

One of the basic concepts of endometriosis has been that it only exists in the presence of ovarian activity with hormone production. In a survey of 350 postmenopausal women, Ranney (1971) found 17 who had active endometriosis, only two of whom had received

11

oestrogen replacement therapy. In 10 of the 17 pain was the major symptom. Djursing et al (1981) from Copenhagen described a case of extensive, active abdominal endometriosis in a postmenopausal woman without any signs of oestrogen activities, while Schram (1978) described a case of endometriosis diagnosed 4 years after 'pelvic clean out'.

Punnonen et al (1980) reported in their series of 20 cases that the average time elapsed since the menopause was 7.3 years after a menopausal average age of 50.3 years. Only one patient in their series had received oestrogen therapy. Some 70% of their postmenopausal patients were obese and they offered an explanation that extraglandular oestrogen formation related to adiposity could explain postmenopausal endometriosis.

Venter et al (1979) reported a case where endometriosis occurred 14 years after hysterectomy and castration with postsurgical oestrogen therapy and where radiotherapy was needed to control the disease—a most unusual situation.

There were eight postmenopausal patients in the Brisbane series and the presenting symptoms and signs are listed in Table 2.4. While

Table 2.4 Postmenopausal patients with endometriosis and coincidental findings

Age	Age at meno- pause	Abdominal pain	Mass	Vaginal bleeding ↑	Weight ↑	Oestrogen replacement therapy	Ovarian ↑	Previous total abdominal hysterec- tomy	Pro- lapse
52	49	+					+		
56	54	+		+	+				
44	41			+	+	+			
51	41			+	+				
49	46	+	+						
43							+		
50	46							+	+
43	41			+			+	+	

it would seem obvious that exogenous oestrogens may reactivate endometriosis after the menopause, in only one of these eight patients had such therapy been employed.

The menarche

The use of the computer made it easy to establish quickly the average age of the menarche in the 717 patients in the endometriosis group as compared with 1000 consecutive patients without endometriosis in the author's practice and the incidence did not show any statistical difference in the two groups. The endometriosis group had an average age of onset of periods of 12.9 years (range 9.3–16.4) and for the non-endometriosis group the average age was 12.6 years.

Prior hormonal contraception

Because so few patients in this series had ever relied upon intrauterine contraceptive devices, there was no point in pursuing this contraceptive factor in the investigation. However, such is the popularity of oral contraceptives in Brisbane that an arbitrary minimal continuous consumption time of 6 months of oral contraceptive therapy was found in 479 patients. The longest duration of continuous oral contraceptive consumption was 11 years to the time of diagnosis. A further 98 patients had taken sequential oral contraceptives continuously for 6 or more months. Thus, 80% (577 out of 717) of the endometriosis patients in the Brisbane series had taken oral contraceptives for at least 6 months suggesting that such action does not reduce the likelihood of developing endometriosis.

This factor becomes more important in the subsequent management of these patients following diagnostic and conservative surgery since there seems little sense in prescribing a preparation postoperatively that is demonstrably of dubious value in the prevention of the disease. Progestogens-only as a form of contraception, or as therapy for dysmenorrhoea or dysfunctional bleeding, had been used in 158 patients in this series, some of whom had also consumed combination or sequential oral contraceptives. This factor did not obviously reduce the likelihood of these patients to suffer from endometriosis although, in fairness, it must be stated that in most of these 158 patients progestogen therapy had not been continuous or prolonged.

Immunosuppressive drug therapy

Because of the author's belief that defective immunocompetence is an important factor in the natural history of endometriosis, a check on the consumption of immunosuppressive agents prior to diagnosis was disappointing in that only seven patients in the series had been on such drug therapy—four had received prednisone for the treatment of asthma, which is a common respiratory complaint in this community, three had received immunosuppressive therapy for ulcerative colitis, Hodgkin's disease, and thyroiditis respectively.

Hereditable factors

Ranney (1970), an indefatigable author on the subject of endometriosis, carried out a review of 350 endometriosis patients in South Dakota and showed that 10% had close female relatives (mother, sister, daughter, cousin, niece) who had required surgery for endometriosis.

Simpson et al (1980) examined the hereditability of endometriosis in a series of 123 patients with histologically proven endometriosis and found that 5.8% of sisters had endometriosis, as did 8.1% of mothers. These workers suggested that endometriosis was several diseases, one form being inherited as the result of a single mutant gene, and others resulting from non-genetic factors or from different genes. They used sister siblings of the husbands of patients with endometriosis as the controls and found an incidence of only 1% in these controls, so that they felt their statistics were satisfactory. They also found that when the clinical picture of endometriosis was examined in affected first degree relatives, it was found to be severe in 61% while it was classified as severe in only 24% in those with no affected first degree relatives.

In the Brisbane series a reliable family history was obtainable in only 538 patients of whom 93 had a sister with endometriosis. In addition, eight mothers in the series subsequently had endometriosis diagnosed in a daughter and there were also two families of four and three daughters respectively where all siblings had surgically proved endometriosis. While these figures suggest a startling familial incidence of about one in five, as opposed to the general incidence in the 6656 patients who are in the practice of one in nine, it must be emphasized that the family histories in many patients are incomplete because of geographic separation etc. However, in view of these facts a heightened awareness of the likelihood of endometriosis existing in mothers, sisters or daughters of patients with surgically proven disease might influence the choice of contraception, the timing of pregnancy, and the extent to which aggressive diagnostic approaches might be appropriate in these women, especially the younger women.

Previous pelvic surgery

The review of the histories of the Brisbane series patients yielded the data shown in Table 2.5. The last patient who had a bilateral adnexectomy previously, had been on oestrogen replacement therapy following surgery by a general surgeon for bilateral ovarian tumours of low-grade malignant potential and she developed endometriosis within a year of surgery and commencing oestrogen replacement therapy.

Table 2.5 Previous pelvic surgery in patients in the Brisbane series

Surgery	Number of patients
D and C	192
Appendicectomy	158
Laparoscopy	64
Tubal occlusion	59
Unilateral ovarian cystectomy	49
Caesarean section	43
Laparotomy	30
Cervical cautery	26
Ventrosuspension	25
Vaginal repair	12
Bilateral ovarian cystectomy	11
Unilateral adnexectomy	10
Total abdominal hysterectomy	5
Vaginal hysterectomy	1
Conization cervix	6
Radical diathermy cervix	5
Myomectomy	4
CO_2 laser therapy cervix	2
Ectopic pregnancy	1
Bilateral adnexectomy	1

In those 59 patients who had had a tubal occlusion previously performed, and in the six with a history of hysterectomy, the possible source of origin of endometriosis cells, and their transtubal transport system, had been interfered with, suggesting some alternative aetiological mechanism in these cases.

Parity

Endometriosis and infertility are commonly thought of as being almost synonymous. In the Brisbane series 392 patients had 1095 pregnancies prior to the surgical diagnosis of endometriosis.

Endometriosis

Correcting the total number of 717 patients for those who had never had coitus (49) and those who had never been married, or in a suitable situation to attempt reproduction (67), the percentage of those having had pregnancies prior to diagnosis is 392 of 601 patients or 65% (Table 2.6).

Table 2.6 Outcome of pregnancy prior to diagnosis of endometriosis

Spontaneous abortion	156 (1 in 7 conceptions)
Ectopic pregnancy	7 (1 in 150 conceptions)
Termination of pregnancy	3
Full-term pregnancy	929

The greatest number of successful pregnancies prior to the diagnosis of endometriosis was 10 and the distribution was as shown in Table 2.7 from which it will be seen that 341 of the 392 patients had a successful pregnancy prior to the diagnosis of endometriosis.

Table 2.7 Parity of 341 parous patients with endometriosis

Parity	Number of patients	Parity	Number of patients
1	66	6	7
2	97	7	2
3	105	8	0
4	54	9	0
5	9	10	1

The abortion rate in the Brisbane series of one in seven conceptions prior to treatment was associated with a one in six incidence after treatment; these figures are at variance with the findings of Wheeler et al (1983) who reported a one in three (34%) incidence in 226 pregnancies prior to diagnosis and treatment of endometriosis that ended in spontaneous first trimester abortion. Following surgery, this incidence was reduced to seven of 76 pregnancies (9%). Termination of pregnancy is only available legally in Brisbane where continuation of the pregnancy will pose a threat to the mother's life so it is not commonly performed.

The incidence of ectopic pregnancy before (one in 150 conceptions) and after (one in 60) diagnosis and treatment of endometriosis is also at variance with the finding of Wheeler & Malinak (1983) who reported that their pretreatment group had an ectopic pregnancy incidence of eight in 64 pregnancies overall, with a curious finding that in a group of patients who were treated and had re-operation without recurrent disease, seven of 16 pregnancies were ectopic. This small fact highlights the importance of a multifactorial aetiology of ectopic pregnancy and the difficulty in relating incidences to a single disease entity. However, the fundamental revelation of this Brisbane experience is that prior pregnancy does not prevent the occurrence or recurrence of endometriosis. Wheeler & Malinak (1983) agree, however, that pregnancy may delay the onset of recurrent endometriosis.

Coincidental disease

A breakdown of the common coincidental disease incidence is shown in Table 2.8 which also compares the incidence in the 5939 patients in the author's practice in whom endometriosis has not been surgically diagnosed.

Table 2.8 Incidence of other diseases in patients with endometriosis and in all other patients

	Endometriosis	No endometriosis
Polycystic ovary disease	259	231
Pelvic inflammatory disease	152	384
Leiomyomata	143	292
Adenomyosis	59	146

The dramatically significant coexistence is with polycystic ovary disease (PCOD) where just over 50% of all patients with PCOD have coexistent endometriosis. Of patients with endometriosis 36% have PCOD. This is different to the findings of Soules et al (1976) who found 58 of 350 (17%) cases of endometriosis were anovulatory, while nine of these 58 (16%) were diagnosed as PCOD. However, they did successfully refute another old axiom about endometriosis— that cyclical ovarian activity is necessary for the production of endometriosis—and their finding that endometriosis and the anovulatory state can coexist is reinforced by the Brisbane series.

It is often difficult to distinguish the damage caused to the internal genitalia, peritoneum, and neighbouring organs by the biological activity of endometriosis deposits from the inflammatory damage resulting from bacterial infection in these organs, especially when there has been no history of acute gynaecological infections. Of course the two disease processes may coexist and the presence of endometriosis must favour significantly more damaging end results when secondary superadded bacterial invasion of these endometriosis deposits occurs.

The coexistence of fibroids and endometriosis is not as dramatic as one of my postgraduate mentors used to predict when he urged female medical undergraduates to marry and reproduce quickly or face a bleak gynaecological future of fibroids and endometriosis. In the light of information presented so far in this book this generalization was invalid on all accounts. There is also a coexistence between fibroids and polycystic ovary disease (112 of 433 patients with fibroids) and all three pathological conditions—endometriosis, fibroids, and polycystic ovary disease—are associated with chronic female sex hormone dysfunction in many patients, but curiously the coincidental incidence of breast disease in the Brisbane series is lower than in the rest of the patients in this practice. Only two of the 717 patients had breast cancer diagnosed while 51 had benign mammary dysplasia. This is notwithstanding the repeated constant diligent search for breast disease in all patients in this practice.

In the last 5 years of the Brisbane series survey, examples of the luteinized unruptured follicle syndrome described by Brosens et al (1978) have been sought. In only 53 patients on direct examination could one confidently confirm the absence of ovulatory stigmata on the luteinized cystic follicle and only 23 of these patients had evidence of endometriosis.

The University of Adelaide investigators, Kerin et al (1983), have prospectively studied 66 regularly cycling women with daily ultrasound and showed an incidence of 4.9% of the luteinized unruptured follicle (LUF) syndrome. Since a recurrence of this phenomenon during prolonged monitoring was relatively rare these workers suggested that the LUF syndrome is really just a biological variable rather than a distinct syndrome.

Another feature of the Brisbane series was the low incidence of associated genital tract congenital anomalies in the 717 cases, there being only four in all. All these patients had partial or complete duplication, none had associated urological abnormalities and two have previously been mentioned in regard to the adolescent endometriosis group.

Vaginal adenosis

Relatively few women in Brisbane have, in the past, been given diethylstilboestrol (DES) in pregnancy and there are only a handful of known cases of DES exposure in utero associated with the subsequent diagnosis of vaginal adenosis, despite much publicity in the lay press. Histologically proven vaginal adenosis without exposure to DES is much more common and coincidentally six of 18 known cases of adenosis also had proven endometriosis. Two of these endometriosis patients were from a group of seven who were known to have been exposed to DES in utero before the twentieth week of development.

Since endometriosis and adenosis are both characterized by ectopically situated glandular epithelium, it seems reasonable to speculate that a similar aetiological mechanism might be responsible for both conditions but no information on such a speculation has yet been published.

Genital tract epithelial dysplasia

The incidence of abnormal cervical cytology in the Brisbane series, 58 of 717 patients, is much higher than the community incidence of seven per 1000 women. The explanation for this may well lie in the fact that the author's main interest is in colposcopy and the role of CO_2 laser therapy in gynaecology, as a consequence of which in the last 4 years of the Brisbane series there had been a relative and absolute increase in the number of patients attending with intra-epithelial neoplasms of the lower genital tract so that the incidence is probably loaded by this factor.

Of the 58 patients, two had herpes simplex type 2 lesions, and 19 had histologically proven human papilloma virus lesions. Perhaps defective immunocompetence leading to these severe inflammatory dysplasias is in some way also responsible for the occurrence of endometriosis in these patients.

Incidence at exploratory surgery

In the past much has been made of the incidence of endometriosis in various socioeconomic groups, private and public hospital patients, and the incidence at laparotomy performed for various reasons. The last 20 years has seen a dramatic change away from laparotomy to laparoscopy for diagnostic procedures and while Williams & Pratt (1977) reported that one-half of the patients involved in the 1000 consecutive laparotomies they reported had endometriosis, I think it unlikely a similar large series of laparotomies will be reviewed in the future.

Much more impressive is the report of Riedel & Semm (1980) that endometriosis was diagnosed in 26% of 5800 laparoscopic examinations of the pelvis. This incidence approximates very nicely with the Brisbane experience where 25% of a total of 1639 patients on whom a laparoscopy was carried out were shown to have endometriosis.

Endometriosis in the male

In 1979 Pinkert et al reported a case of endometriosis of the urinary bladder in a male who had been treated with oestrogen for several years following radical prostatectomy and orchidectomy for prostatic cancer. In the following year Schrodt et al (1980) reported a further case of a 73-year-old male who had an adenocarcinoma of the prostate for which he had been given oestrogen therapy for 5 years before endometriotic tissue, involving the right urethro-vesical junction, was removed. The seemingly incredible ability of synthetic oestrogens to induce such a dramatic and profound histological change in the male urinary tract epithelium may provoke further research into the possible causal relationship between exogenous oestrogens (as ingested in oral contraceptive pills) and endometriosis in females.

Endometriosis in non-human primates

Endometriosis has been reported in the non-human primates. The non-appearance of endometriosis in other animals is probably related to the fact that they do not have cyclical menstrual periods. The first report of endometriosis in a monkey was published in 1929 (Fraser 1929) and since then a number of cases has been reported in non-human primates. In addition to rhesus monkeys the disease has been noted in cynomolgus monkeys, baboons, pigtail macaques and African green monkeys.

As well as probably having a spontaneous aetiology, non-human primate endometriosis may also be associated with prior exposure to irradiation, hysterectomy, deliberate implantation of endometrial tissue excised from the uterine lining and following experimental surgery (Telinde & Scott 1950). In monkeys the disease is characterized by dysmenorrhoea, menorrhagia, irregular menstrual cycles and infertility. More extensive disease may cause obstruction of the ureters, small intestine, large intestine, and death as a result of such obstruction, or following haemorrhage into the abdominal cavity.

The gross and histological features of endometriosis in monkeys and women are comparable and non-human primates probably suffer more extensive abdominal cavity fibrous adhesions.

In an autopsy series including 821 adult female non-human primates, McClure (1979) reported 16 cases of endometriosis and/or adenomyosis—an overall incidence of 1.9%. He found that 12 cases occurred in rhesus monkeys, two in pigtail macaques, one in an African green monkey and one in a gelada baboon. The overall incidence for autopsied adult females of each species was 5.6% (12 out of 212) for rhesus; 6.6% (two out of 30) for pigtail macaques; 14.2% (one out of seven) for African green monkeys and 14.2% (one out of seven) for gelada baboons. In this autopsy series endometriosis was not seen in 42 adult female great apes, 392 adult female New World monkeys, or in 47 adult female prosimians.

The approximate age of affected females ranged from 6 to 21 years and five of the 12 rhesus monkeys had a history of irradiation exposure. One African green monkey had received an oestrogen implant 3 years prior to death and one rhesus monkey was oophorectomized 7 years prior to death and had received oestrogen implants 1, 2 and 6 years following removal of the ovaries. None of the animals with endometriosis or adenomyosis had had a hysterotomy.

Both endometriosis and adenomyosis were present in nine of the 16 cases; two had early adenomyosis and in five, only extrauterine lesions were present with no evidence of adenomyosis. McClure reported that he had seen one case where an animal had adenomyosis and endometriosis where the adenomyosis appeared to be the more extensive lesion in that the degree of uterine distortion was disproportionately large compared to the extrauterine lesions. The uterine enlargement, in fact, had been so great as to cause ureteric obstruction. McClure found that the commonest sites for ectopic endometrium included the uterine serosa and adjacent structures, ovaries, mesentery and wall of the colon. He reported that occasionally endometriotic nodules were seen on the serosa of the bladder, spleen and liver. Schiffer et al (1984) reported a case of endometriosis in a rhesus monkey where an acute haemoperitoneum had been associated with extensive endometriosis involving the uterine surface, bowel and surface of most of the visceral organs especially the liver. These workers compared the onset of haemorrhage in their monkey patients at the time of menstruation with the usual perimenstrual haemorrhage that occurs with human females with endometriosis. In both species the ectopic endometrial tissue is highly vascularized at this time of the menstrual cycle and in primates avulsion or rupture of large cysts is much more likely than in humans. It is of interest to note that these workers also described a history of dysmenorrhoea in primates as being evidenced by cyclical depression and anorexia, features not unknown in human females.

The close similiarity of the disease process in these two species would indicate that further investigation of the use of non-human primates as experimental models for researching the aetiology, natural history, pathological process and response to various therapeutic modalities in endometriosis is obviously indicated.

Doubtless in some parts of the world animal lovers will react to this suggestion in horror, but the fact that the disease occurs spontaneously in non-human primates could be used as justification for such research on the basis that it may, in the long run, improve the quality of life for these animals as well as for human female sufferers.

The role of ovarian steroids in the form of silastic implants of oestradiol and/or progesterone—in the initiation, maintenance, and suppression of endometriosis in female cynomolgus monkeys—has already been researched by DiZerega et al (1980). They found that, although endometrial transplants on peritoneum required no steroid supplementation for initiation of endometriosis, maintenance depended on oestradiol or progesterone, alone or together. It is to be hoped that more work of this nature will be forthcoming in the future.

REFERENCES

Brosens I A, Konincks P, Corveleyn P A 1978 A study of plasma progesterone, oestradiol 17β, prolactin, LH levels, and the luteal phase appearance of the ovaries in patients with endometriosis and infertility. British Journal of Obstetrics and Gynaecology 85:246–250

Chatman D L 1976 Endometriosis in the black woman. American Journal of Obstetrics and Gynecology 125:7 987–989

Chatman D L, Ward A B 1982 Endometriosis in adolescents. Journal of Reproductive Medicine 27:3 156–160

DiZerega G S, Barber D L, Hodgen G T 1980 Endometriosis: role of ovarian steroids in initiation, maintenance and suppression. Fertility and Sterility 33:649–653

Djursing H, Peterson K, Weberg E 1981 Symptomatic post menopausal endometriosis. Acta Obstetrica et Gynaecologica Scandinavica 60:529–530

Ekwempu C C, Harrison K A 1979 Endometriosis among the Hausa-Fulani population of Nigeria. Tropical Geographic Medicine 31:2 201–205

Fraser A D 1929 Ectopic endometrium in a macacus rhesus. Journal of Obstetrics and Gynaecology of the British Commonwealth 36:590–591

Goldstein D P, de Cholnoky C, Emans S J, Leventhall J M 1980 Laparoscopy in the management of pelvic pain in adolescents. Journal of Reproductive Medicine 24:6 251–256

Jansen R P S 1982 Pelvic surgery in young women. Medical Journal of Australia 1:525–526

Kerin J F, Kirby L, Morris D, McEvoy M, Ward B, Cox L 1983 Incidence of the luteinized unruptured follicle phenomenon in cycling women. Fertility and Sterility 40:620–626

McClure H M 1979 Endometriosis. In: Andrews E J, Ward B C, Altman N H (eds) Spontaneous animal models of human disease. Academic Press Inc, New York vol 1, p 215–218

Miyazawa K 1976 Incidence of endometriosis among Japanese women. Obstetrics and Gynecology 48:407–409

Pinkert T, Catlow L E, Strauss R 1979 Endometriosis in the urinary bladder in a man with prostatic cancer. Cancer 43:1562–1567

Punnonen R, Klemi P J, Nikkanen U 1980 Postmenopausal endometriosis. European Journal of Obstetrics, Gynecology and Reproductive Biology 11:195–200

Ranney B 1970 Endometriosis IV: hereditary tendency. Obstetrics and Gynecology 37:5 734–737

Ranney B 1971 Endometriosis III: complete operations. American Journal of Obstetrics and Gynecology 109:1137–1144

Riedel H, Semm K 1980 Clinical aspects of endometriosis externa. Zentralblatt für Gynaekologie 102:981–989

Schiffer S P, Cary C J, Peter G K, Cohen B J 1984 Haemoperitoneum associated with endometriosis in a rhesus monkey. Journal of the American Veterinary Medicine Association 185:1375–1377

Schifrin B S, Erez S, Morre J G 1973 Teenage endometriosis. American Journal of Obstetrics and Gynecology 116:973–980

Schram J D 1978 Endometriosis after pelvic cleanout. Southern Medical Journal 71:1414–1420

Schrodt G R, Alcorn M O, Ibanez J 1980 Endometriosis of the male urinary system: a case report. Journal of Urology 124:722–723

Simpson J C, Elias S, Malinak L R, Buttram V C Jr 1980 Hereditable aspects of endometriosis I: genetic studies. American Journal of Obstetrics and Gynecology 137:327–331

Soules M R, Malinak L R, Bury R, Poindexter H 1976 Endometriosis and anovulation: a coexisting problem in the infertile female. American Journal of Obstetrics and Gynecology 125:3 412–417

TeLinde R W, Scott R B 1950 Experimental endometriosis. American Journal of Obstetrics and Gynecology 60:1147–1173

Venter P F, Anderson J D, Van Velden D J 1979 Postmenopausal endometriosis: a case report. South African Medical Journal 56:1136–1138

Wheeler J M, Johnston B M, Malinak L R 1983 The relationship of endometriosis to spontaneous abortion. Fertility and Sterility 39:656–660

Wheeler J M, Malinak L R 1983 Recurrent endometriosis: incidence management and prognosis. American Journal of Obstetrics and Gynecology 146:247–253

Williams T J, Pratt J R 1977 Endometriosis in 1000 consecutive coeliotomies: evidence and management. American Journal of Obstetrics and Gynecology 129:245–250

3

Aetiology and pathogenesis

There are so many theories as to the aetiology of endometriosis that obviously no single theory covers all clinical presentations of the disease. Either there are multiple disease processes each with a unique aetiology, or one disease process with a multifactorial aetiology. Hereditable factors were considered in the discussion of the epidemiology of endometriosis and a brief review of the more traditional aetiological theories is in order before considering more contemporary propositions.

Since 1860 when Rokitansky first described the disease entity now known as endometriosis (Dewhurst 1981), the theories of origin were, until recently, related to the mechanics of the development of the disease. Von Recklinghausen (1885) originally proposed a theory of development in embryonic tissue of wolffian origin while Cullen (1896) suggested that such development more likely took place in embryonic tissue of mullerian origin. Iwanhof (1898) first suggested the possibility of metaplasia of serosal peritoneum, while Meyer (1903) and others further developed this hypothesis and suggested that under the influence of hormones or inflammation, pelvic peritoneum might form tubular invaginations which sink progressively deeper into neighbouring organs while simultaneously transforming flattened peritoneal endothelium into columnar epithelium, having the glandular appearance of endometrial tissue, now ectopically located. Pick (1905) suggested a similar process involving the germinal epithelium of the ovary.

In 1980 El-Mahgoub & Yaseen described a case that they believed proved the coelomic metaplasia theory because their patient had primary amenorrhoea and endometriosis. It would seem much more logical to suggest that patients with congenital absence of the uterus (endometrium) and proven endometriosis would prove the coelomic

24

metaplasia theory, but no such cases have been found in the literature.

The easiest causal theory to understand—and to explain to patients—is that of Sampson who, in 1922, first postulated that retrograde menstruation with transtubal migration of viable, shed endometrial cells and subsequent successful attachment and implantation with continuing biological function, produced endometriosis. Of course this theory does not take into account the fact that not every woman with retrograde menstruation develops endometriosis; of 85 women having a laparoscopic examination during menstruation in the Brisbane series, 80 showed evidence of retrograde menstruation, but only 15 had endometriosis.

Sampson's theory also did not account for those in whom the disease appears for the first time after removal of the source of endometrial cells by hysterectomy or following obstruction to retrograde menstruation by bilateral tubal obstruction, either surgically induced for sterilization purposes, or by disease process.

Halban (1924) and Sampson also offered a further explanation that endolymphatic spread could account for extrapelvic endometriosis and this was confirmed by Javert (1951), while Navrital and Kramer (1936) suggested vascular embolization as a cause of remote extragenital location of endometriosis deposits.

When TeLinde and Scott (1951) applied Sampson's theory of retrograde menstruation to primates in an experimental situation, they found uterine retroversion favoured the production of endometriosis.

A rarely mentioned paper from New Zealand (McVeigh 1955) postulated an interesting theory based on histological morphology. McVeigh believed that those ova released at ovulation and not entrapped by tubal fimbria, literally fell by the wayside into the pouch of Douglas. He believed that the corona radiata (cumulus) enveloping the developing ovum in the follicle, could separate readily from the follicle and escape with the ovum at ovulation. Having the same morphological origin as endometrial cells, he believed that under certain unspecified hormonal conditions, the cumulus could produce ectopically located endometrial cells and endometriosis. Since the advent of high technology and in vitro fertilization, the separation of the cumulus from the ovum has become a real possibility rather than a theoretical proposition so another antique speculative theory may be less speculative than originally thought.

More contemporary factors concerning the aetiology of endometriosis may be considered quite appropriately under the following headings:

1. Ovarian morphology and function
2. Immunology
3. The role of prostaglandins
4. Endocrine factors from the hypothalmic-pituitary-ovarian axis
5. Mechanical implantation factors

Ovarian morphology and function

It is no longer accepted that endometriosis can only coexist with normal ovulatory ovarian function. The very high coincidence of polycystic ovary disease (PCOD) and endometriosis in the Brisbane series highlights this fact. The phenomenon of luteinization of an unruptured ovarian follicle has attracted much interest since Jewelewicz (1975) described this syndrome wherein the oocyte remains trapped in a ripened follicle which fails to rupture. The follicle undergoes orthodox luteinization producing progesterone which in turn alters the endometrium to a secretory pattern, thus mimicking a normal ovulatory potentially fertile pattern of behaviour associated with a fertile type basal temperature chart. Absence of a visible stoma in the luteinized structure from which the ovum could have been released is the laparoscopic criterion for the diagnosis of this condition. Since the luteinized unruptured follicle (LUF) syndrome was reported in as many as 79% of women with endometriosis by Brosens et al (1978) it has been carefully sought at laparoscopy and laparotomy by the author, and proved elusive.

It could be that the LUF syndrome is the primary abnormality resulting in infertility which then predisposes to the initiation and continuation of endometriosis, so that the traditional thinking that endometriosis causes infertility may in fact be true in reverse—more accurately infertility leads to endometriosis. The concept of the LUF syndrome has been supported by Koninckx et al (1978) and by their research into the volume and biochemical content of peritoneal fluids in patients with and without the LUF syndrome as determined by the presence or absence of ovarian ovulatory stigmata. Women with ovulatory stigmata had high concentrations of 17-β-oestradiol and progesterone for at least 6 days post ovulation. Women without ovulatory stigmata had barely elevated steroid hormone concentrations during the early luteal phase except when the corpus luteum was cystic. These workers claim steroid hormone levels in peritoneal fluid are a reflection of ovarian exudation, and reach much higher levels than in the blood, so that a more sensitive indication of steroid production can be obtained from peritoneal fluid rather than from peripheral blood. The volume of peritoneal fluid, which expands with increased ovarian function, reaches a peak at ovulation and then falls away progressively to menstruation. It is postulated that in the LUF syndrome the decreased volume of peritoneal fluid contains very reduced levels of sex steroid hormones and thus the required inhibiting effect of these ovarian steroid hormones to prevent transtubally regurgitated shed endometrial cells at menstruation from implanting in the peritoneal surface is absent.

Donnez et al (1983) have advocated peritoneal fluid aspiration and sampling for steroid hormone assay to diagnose the LUF syndrome which, according to Devroey et al (1983) is very amenable to gonadotrophin therapy. Koninckx et al (1980a) noted no significant difference in the volume of peritoneal fluid in women with or without endometriosis, but Drake et al (1980) claimed that throughout the menstrual cycle there was a considerable increase in peritoneal fluid production in endometriosis and they, in contradistinction to Koninckx et al, found that more severe endometriosis produced a more significantly increased volume of peritoneal fluid.

Dmowski et al (1980) disputed the hypothesis of the Belgian workers Koninckx et al that the LUF syndrome may be the cause of infertility in women with endometriosis. In particular they reported a significant difference in the incidence of the LUF syndrome in the control groups in their own studies, those of the Belgian workers, and those of Marik & Hulka (1978). A research team from the University of Adelaide in Australia has produced an ultrasound study of the ovary in the detection of the LUF syndrome (Kerin et al 1983). These workers noted the indirect evidence that this syndrome may be more common in women with endometriosis (Brosens et al 1978); that it could be more common in unexplained infertility (Koninckx et al 1978, Marik & Hulka 1978), and following ovulation induction with clomiphene citrate (Coulam et al 1982). They noted the direct evidence obtained at laparoscopic evaluation by the Belgian workers in 1980 and Marik & Hulka 1978, that the LUF syndrome could also be diagnosed in a proportion of apparently ovulatory cycles.

The Adelaide study established an incidence of 4.9% of the LUF syndrome in a population of 66 regularly cycling females and because of its infrequent recurrence in subsequent monitored cycles, these workers preferred to consider the LUF syndrome as an isolated phenomenon rather than a syndrome. They found no increased incidence of the phenomenon in preliminary studies of five women with proven endometriosis monitored over five cycles.

Researching the role of ovarian steroids in the initiation, maintenance, and suppression of endometriosis in cynomolgus monkeys DiZerega et al (1981) found that while initiation of endometriosis could be independent of the steroids, maintenance of endometriotic plaques was highly dependent on both oestrogen and progesterone.

A number of important contemporary studies into the problems of endometriosis were presented to the fortieth annual meeting of the American Fertility Society at New Orleans, Louisiana in April 1984.

Gibbons et al (1984) presented the results of a study of the incidence of the LUF syndrome in a population of infertile women using ultrasound screening. Screening 153 women over 263 cycles they found that 14 (9.2%) showed the syndrome. Laparoscopic evaluation of these 14 patients showed that five had endometriosis— this incidence being no greater than that observed in the overall infertile population. In a group of clomiphene-stimulated patients they found the incidence of the LUF syndrome was 9.6% compared with 9% in the untreated group. They also found that an injection of 5000 units of human chorionic gonadotrophin invariably produced ovulation in patients with the LUF syndrome as determined by ultrasound screening changes. They concluded that endometriosis is not more prevalent in the group of infertile patients showing LUF criteria.

A group of workers in Helsinki, Liukkonen et al (1984) also employed ultrasound to evaluate the diagnosis of the LUF syndrome in 37 women with unexplained infertility, monitoring over two to three menstrual cycles. Analysis of the results obtained in over 100 cycles, revealed 57 incidences of the LUF syndrome, 33 incidences of collapsed follicle, and 10 cases of anovulation. Of the 57 examples of the LUF syndrome, 25 women were further evaluated by laparoscopy or laparotomy during day 16 to 18 of the third cycle. Eighteen of the 21 women with ultrasound diagnosis of LUF showed a corpus luteum without ovulatory stigmata, but three showed ovulatory stigmatas so had to be considered as false positive ultrasound diagnoses of LUF. Endometriosis was diagnosed at operation in seven women of whom five also had the LUF syndrome. The syndrome occurred in only 34% of the patients in three consecutive cycles as diagnosed by ultrasound.

These findings would suggest that the uncommon detection of the LUF syndrome in the Brisbane series since the author became aware of its existence some 5 years ago is probably not exceptional and that the concept of the Adelaide workers that this is a transient phenomenon rather than a definite ongoing syndrome, is probably correct. This is not to say, however, that the theoretical description of Brosens and his co-workers of how the disturbed reduced ovarian steroidogenesis associated with LUF—even if only transient—can produce the appropriate climate for endometriosis to develop, is invalid.

Immunological considerations

The constant conundrum in the development of endometriosis is 'why does not every menstruating female develop endometriosis?' The possibility of some women having a genetic predisposition to this disease was considered in the epidemiological section. The incidence in the Brisbane series of two families where four and three siblings in each family had endometriosis with a 100% sibling incidence suggests support for this theory.

Of equal importance is the question of altered immunocompetence. While a report from Brekken & Massey (1980) of a heart transplant patient developing an endometriotic mass 3 years after her transplant, demonstrated the dramatically obvious possible role of immunosuppression in the development of endometriosis, it is surprising that there have not been more reported cases of endometriosis in immunosuppressed menstruating females who have received, for instance, renal transplants—a not uncommon surgical procedure at the present time. A previous history of immune-status altering drugs was uncommon in the Brisbane series.

The presence of macrophages in the peritoneum of patients with endometriosis has been examined by several teams and variable significance attributed to this finding. Muscato et al (1982) found increased numbers of peritoneal macrophages present in women with endometriosis and these macrophages in infertile women with endometriosis, phagocytosed more normal sperm in vitro than macrophages from normal fertile women, or infertile women without endometriosis.

Halme et al (1983) considered the increased pelvic macrophage activity of infertile women with endometriosis. They collected pelvic fluid from 66 women at either diagnostic laparoscopy for evaluation of infertility including patients with mild endometriosis, or at laparoscopic tubal occlusion. The cellular fraction was separated out (mainly macrophages) and stained for peritoneal irritants (acid phosphatase and myeloperoxidase). The fluid fraction was analysed for acid phosphatase, neutral protease and extractable prostaglandins PGE_2 and $PGF_{2\alpha}$.

Their findings showed no significant difference in the prostanoid fraction between groups of patients but a high proportion of the macrophages in the mild endometriosis patients showed positive acid phosphatase staining (46%) compared with the group of normal fertility (15%) and the pelvic fluid analysis for the mild endometriosis patients showed a higher acid phosphatase and neutral protease activity than in non-endometriosis patients of proven fertility.

These findings suggest that activation of macrophages and release of active substances into the peritoneal fluid may contribute to infertility in endometriosis. Obviously more work needs to be done with regard to macrophages and endometriosis.

Dmowski et al (1981) showed that rhesus monkeys with spontaneous endometriosis had an altered cellular immune response to autologous antigens. They suggested that although such animals were demonstrated to be immunocompetent in general, they showed in particular a diminished cell-mediated response to autologous endometrial antigens. Their conclusion was that endometrial cells translocated from their normal location might only implant ectopically in women with a specific cell-mediated immunity defect.

Weed & Arquembourg (1980) considered the possibility that endometriosis could produce an autoimmune response in the victim, in turn producing infertility, and pointed out that endometriosis often occurs in women of previously proven fertility as was shown dramatically in the Brisbane series. Weed & Arquembourg explained that autoimmune mechanisms are present in the mullerian system to combat foreign antigens. Various levels of the reproductive system, excepting the ectocervix, secrete IgA, IgG, IgM immunoglobulins. Complement, a complex arrangement of interacting proteins, interacts with immunoglobulins to complete the antibody response. Humoral antibodies are produced when plasma cells derived from B lymphocytes and sensitized as immunocytes, react with an antigen. The complement system should be present from birth but may be congenitally absent, or depleted by active disease, and only return to normal when disease is inactivated. The author wonders whether oral contraceptives do not, in some way, interfere with the complement system perhaps thus making women more prone to the development of endometriosis.

The complement system involves a cascade of 11 discrete proteins (Weed & Arquembourg 1980) in a classic sequence following activation by antigen–antibody response, and complement, C3, is deposited on target cells destroying them or altering their function. Endometriosis, according to Weed & Arquembourg, creates an antigen of the host's own endometrial cells which are identified as 'foreign' by the host, and while the nature of the antigen has not been identified, the effects of the antibody have been to precipitate the deposition of complement around the endometrial glands, possibly causing infertility by rejection of early embryonic implantation, or by interference with sperm passage.

This could also explain the observation of in vitro fertilization workers that given optimal circumstances and successful ovum pick-up in endometriosis patients, successful outcome from in vitro fertilization and embryo transfer seems to be more elusive than for other infertile women.

The fact that postulated autoimmune reactions can be reversed with surgical excision of endometriosis, or prolonged ovarian suppression, suggests that it must be a weak autoimmune system. Bartosic et al (1984) showed that 22 of 35 patients with endometriosis had either C3 or C4 complement in the uterine endometrium—11 in proliferative endometrium and 11 in secretory endometrium. They also reported that of four patients with stage I endometriosis who became pregnant, none had C complement in the endometrium. They also found that C3 or C4 were present in the endometrium in 13 of 17 patients with pelvic inflammatory disease. Their hypothesis was that the mechanism for infertility in endometriosis patients positive for C3 or C4 is a 'cytolytic anti-implantation effect' induced by the presence of complement.

Badaway et al (1984) found, by using sophisticated immunoassays and immunoelectrophoresis studies, that serum and peritoneal fluid of 23 patients with endometriosis showed significantly higher concentrations of C3 and C4 than a control group of women without endometriosis. This area of research into immunology and endometriosis obviously will be explored further in the future.

However, one might ask again why does this not affect all women, all women with infertility, or all women with endometriosis? Is there a genetic factor involved as well?

Role of prostaglandins in endometriosis

Prostaglandin secretion from uterus and ovary usually exhibits a cyclical pattern varying in relation to the menstrual hormone production pattern. Prostaglandin synthesis is stimulated by the combined effect of oestradiol and progesterone but does not reach high levels unless the plasma progesterone level is significantly elevated. This effect of plasma progesterone is probably related to binding and storage of prostaglandin in endometrial tissue and normal endometrium contains relatively large quantities of prostaglandin ($PGF_{2\alpha}$) in the secretory phase. Peristalsis and cilial activity in the fallopian tube (which have an important effect on ovum transplant) are directly influenced by the prostaglandins and the fallopian tube contains both PGE and $PGF_{2\alpha}$.

While Drake et al (1981) have shown elevated levels of prostaglandin metabolites (thromboxane B2 and 6-keto-prostaglandin F) in peritoneal fluid of women with endometriosis, Rock et al (1982) have not been able to confirm these findings in fluid obtained in the proliferative phase of the cycle. Unidentified factors in the peritoneal fluid have been implicated by the fact that peritoneal fluid collected from endometriosis patients in the luteal phase significantly reduces sperm survival time in vitro (Elstein & Filho 1980) and one wonders if macrophages might be important in this regard.

Ylikorkala & Tenhunen (1984) have determined follicular fluid prostaglandin levels in a group of patients—17 with endometriosis, a control group of 17 with tubal occlusion and normal ovaries, and five with induced ovarian hyperstimulation—by laparoscopically aspirating follicles and measuring prostaglandin metabolites by radioimmunoassay. They found no difference in the concentrations, and similar results in the three groups, so while these prostanoids are produced in vivo by the follicle, they may have no primary significance in either ovulation or endometriosis.

On the other hand, Moon et al (1981) measured the prostaglandin concentration of ovarian tissue, with or without endometriosis, compared with uterine endometrium prostaglandin levels in five patients with endometriosis. Their study group included one patient in whom they could compare the contents of an endometriotic cyst with a follicular cyst. The results strongly indicated that ectopic endometrium in endometriosis contains higher levels of PGF than the stroma of a normal ovary, than normal endometrium, and than a follicle cyst in the same patient. They suggest that the role of PGF in infertility is by luteolysis and interference with tubal motility while its influence on endometrial and vascular contractility may produce the pain of endometriotic dysmenorrhoea.

Weed (1980) saw that antiprostaglandin agents could have a useful role in the treatment of endometriosis on the basis that increased dysmenorrhoea in endometriosis is due to increased PGF production from endometriotic implants, and in response to damage and inflammation caused by the direct effect of these implants in their ectopic location.

Olive et al (1982) believe that the higher incidence of spontaneous abortion in endometriosis sufferers is related to prostaglandin excess produced by endometrial implants and that the presence of endometriomata may also irritate and produce resulting uterine spasms sufficient to disrupt a pregnancy.

Hypothalamo-pituitary-ovarian axis factors

A. Endometriosis and hyperprolactinaemic galactorrhoea

It has been postulated that endometriosis is associated with emotional stress especially when infertility is a complication (Koninckx & Brosens 1982). It is also possible that this stress acting through the hypothalamo-pituitary-ovarian axis, produces the increased prolactin secretion in endometriosis victims found by Muse et al (1982). Their findings were at variance with those of Hirschowitz et al (1978) who described a new syndrome of endometriosis and galactorrhoea in eight women, seven of whom had normal prolactin levels. They suggested galactorrhoea in the female with normal menses should intimate underlying endometriosis especially if dysmenorrhoea was a dominant symptom, but the association seems speculative.

Hyperprolactinaemia in infertility is certainly understandable and, as happened in both the Brisbane series patients with galactorrhoea, infertility and endometriosis, the use of bromocriptine seemed to cure the galactorrhoea and infertility if not the endometriosis. Since all patients in the Brisbane series have had repeated and regular breast examinations, and since in the other patients there were many instances of inappropriate lactation without evidence of endometriosis, it is believed that the relationship between galactorrhoea and endometriosis is nothing more than coincident.

B. Endometriosis and luteal inadequacy

Cheesman et al (1982) studied the concentrations of luteinizing hormone (LH), pregnanediol-3 (PGD), -glucuronide and oestriol-16-glucuronide in daily morning urine specimens from 53 infertile women. In 26 of 29 with various degrees of proven endometriosis, two distinct LH peaks were found 2 or 3 days apart. Those patients with the most severe forms of endometriosis had LH peaks separated by up to 3 days and luteal function was shorter than usual as the maximum PGD concentration was reached. This did not occur until the time of the second peak. It would appear from data on LH production that there is an inappropriate feedback mechanism operative in patients with endometriosis.

There are of course those who dispute the significance of luteal inadequacy in endometriosis but the striking coincidental finding of polycystic ovary disease in patients with endometriosis the Brisbane series has to be significant in the pathogenesis of both disease processes.

C. Polycystic ovary disease

In 259 of 717 patients in the Brisbane series, PCOD was a coincidental finding as was the fact that overall in this practice endometriosis occurred in 50% of patients with PCOD. Apart from the association of each disease entity with infertility there does not seem to be much in common between the two.

Long before Stein and Leventhal read their milestone paper on PCOD to the Central Association of Obstetricians & Gynaecologists in November 1934 at New Orleans, the entity had been surgically identified and those cases showing bilateral multicystic ovaries with pearly white sclerotic capsules were labelled sclerotic disease of the ovary. Katz et al (1978) noted that Waldow in 1895 was the first to recommend ovarian wedge resection-type surgery for this condition rather than the previously recommended oophorectomy. In 1935 Stein & Leventhal published their paper on amenorrhoea associated with bilateral polycystic ovaries and in reporting the serendipidous finding that wedge resection cured amenorrhoea in six of their seven cases, they quite by chance, introduced what was to become in some hands a much abused and overused gynaecological surgical procedure—wedge resection of the ovary. They also gave their names to a syndrome but this is no longer appropriate since there are so many variations on the original theme of anovulatory infertility, menstrual disorders, hirsutism, obesity, bilateral polycystic ovaries, that it is now more usual to use the expression Polycystic Ovary Disease or PCO syndrome. The contemporary variable clinical picture includes all forms of menstrual disturbance from perimenarchial primary amenorrhoea to oligomenorrhoea; evidence of androgen excess (hirsutism, sebaceous skin disorders and acne); variable weight patterns usually with a tendency to obesity, again often starting soon after puberty, and the one constant feature is the presence of polycystic ovaries which may or may not be enlarged.

Biggs (1981) reviewed the then current status of PCOD and mentioned the great variability in acceptable histological features of this condition, and the confusion about hormone assays early in the history of the disease. He noted, however, that with the use of radioimmunoassay techniques some blood levels of hormone production had been freely defined in PCOD. For instance it can be concluded that LH levels are higher than normal, mid-cycle LH peak is absent, and there is a pattern of irregular fluctuation about a raised base line; follicle stimulating hormone (FSH) levels are similar to those in normal women; the oestrone level is higher than in normal females and higher than the levels of oestradiol, as is more usually seen after the menopause, and this has been attributed to the peripheral conversion of androstenedione to oestradiol.

Biggs noted that in two studies from LaJolla, California, and Birmingham, England, oestradiol levels were similar in PCOD and normal women in the United States series, and higher in women with PCOD in the United Kingdom series. He, however, drew attention to the fact that comparisons of oestradiol levels in these situations depend very much on the stage of the cycle at which samples are assayed. Total oestrogen levels were raised in PCOD; testosterone was significantly higher than normal and androstenedione had much higher and more pronounced levels in PCOD than even testosterone. Biggs & Thomas (1981) determined by a selective slice and culture technique utilizing wedge resection specimens that androstenedione and oestriol were produced principally by the ovarian cortex with very little contribution from the medullary cells.

Enzyme deficiencies in PCOD

Several varieties of cellular enzyme disorder have been identified in PCOD: defective aromatization of steroids after the oxygenation stage of 19 methyl group; deficiency of 3β-OH steroid dehydrogenase;

and reduced 17-hydroxylase activity. Are these genetically acquired deficiencies or transient aberrations? Vaitukaitis (1983) suggests PCOD may be an X-linked dominant inherited disorder.

Hormonal inter-relationships in PCOD

The raised LH level of PCOD is associated with increased sensitivity of gonadotrophin cell LH secretion to gonadotrophin-releasing hormone (GnRH) and there is a similar FSH response to GnRH. LH is mainly responsible for theca cell stimulation and FSH for granulosa cell stimulation and oestradiol production in ovarian follicles. The small follicle cysts in PCOD have been shown to be deficient in aromatase activity normally stimulated by FSH.

FSH and LH have complementary roles in follicular development. In PCOD, with higher LH levels, the balance is disturbed and excessive theca cell stimulation occurs with increased androgen production. The follicles so involved, not receiving an LH surge as in an ordinary ovulatory cycle, enlarge and persist as cysts averaging around 8 mm in diameter, multiple in number, and all of similar size. The increased androgen production in PCOD in turn leads to increased peripheral conversion of androstenedione to testosterone and some is also converted to oestrone. This raises the total circulating oestrogen levels above normal and may lead to altered sensitivity of pituitary production of LH in response to GnRH stimulation, in turn producing a self-perpetuating cycle of action and response.

Zumhoff et al (1983) investigated possible abnormalities of CNS regulation of LH secretion in PCOD by determining plasma LH levels in five teenagers with PCOD over a 24-h period. They found in normal postpubertal girls there was a daily surge of LH coterminous with their nocturnal sleep period, but in four of the PCOD teenagers LH surges occurred 7–8 hours later in the daytime than normal. This chronobiological disturbance only involved LH, not cortisol nor prolactin, and only occurred in four of the five subjects. From the author's personal experience of sharing some of his life with three teenage daughters in the same age group as the Zumhoff study group (13–16), it is suggested that two factors may have been overlooked by Zumhoff et al: first, all postpubertal girls have some phases of PCO activity as a normal variant in the process of hypothalamo-pituitary-ovarian maturation in the postpubertal phase; and second, the notion of a routine regular sleep pattern in girls of this age would seem to be quite unusual!

Vaitukaitis (1983) has suggested a hypothalamic defect possibly related to a functional depletion of dopamine within the hypothalamic nuclei as a possible aetiology for PCOD but this is an area of ongoing research.

In obese patients the conversion of androstenedione peripherally to oestrone is facilitated by adipocytes and this unopposed oestrogen production can lead to secondary disease problems; endometrial hyperplasia and neoplasia, ovarian tumours, breast disease, and hypertension, as well as perpetuating the obesity and emotional problems associated with PCOD.

Management of PCOD

For many years the management was surgical. Indeed Hjortrup et al as recently as 1983 reported that 26 of 29 patients with PCOD having wedge resections and followed up for up to 9 years, had established normal menstrual patterns with a 100% pregnancy rate in 10 patients wishing to conceive. Eight of the nine patients who were obese preoperatively and who had normal menstrual cycles postoperatively showed a major weight loss after wedge resection, while none of those who remained oligomenorrhoeic after operation lost weight. Hirsutism was not cured by wedge resection. On the other hand, Gjönnaess (1984) demonstrated a neat laparoscopic technique with systematic ovarian capsular electrocautery which produced ovulation in 92% of 62 patients within 3 months of operation and there was a 69% pregnancy rate in those who were infertile, improving to 80% when those patients shown to be sensitive to clomiphene were included.

The standard non-surgical treatment for PCOD for many years has been to use antioestrogenic preparations to induce ovulation and break the cycle of disturbed hormonal activity. This was especially important where infertility was a problem. Clomiphene citrate used in doses from 50 to 200 mg daily for 5 days, with or without human chorionic gonadotrophin injections from 3000–9000 IU mid-cycle, has produced excellent results, but there is always some 10–20% of patients who do not respond to this therapy. For these Gjönnaess suggests his technique is of value where non-surgical methods have failed to produce ovulation. Where open operation is indicated, and because of the extra potential threats to infertility following open surgery, modified CO_2 laser wedge resection technique as demonstrated by Chong & Baggish (1984) would seem to have the most favourable and auspicious prognostic advantages combining surgical sophistication and high technology with a predictable old time remedial attack.

Of course there are many patients with PCOD and endometriosis who are not bothered by infertility and for whom, in fact, ovulation induction would be mischievous.

Androgenic symptoms can be reversed by simple appropriate suppressive therapy, for example dexamethasone 0.5 mg daily for 60–90 days.

For those patients in whom excessive oestrogen activity is a problem, correction with progestogens is very effective and in this regard medroxyprogesterone acetate is a most useful preparation in the treatment of both PCOD and endometriosis as will be discussed in Chapter 6.

Mechanical implantation factors

Reports of endometriosis occurring in episiotomy scars (Hambrick et al 1979) and along amniocentesis needle tracks (Kaunitz & di Sant'agnese 1979) and in surgical scars are not rare. One consequence of the relatively high Caesarean section rate in some obstetric units, it is believed, will be an increase in the number of women presenting with post-Caesarean adenomyosis and endometriosis associated with uterine scarring. Already the Brisbane series includes a number of patients in whom extensive endometriosis has been discovered 1–10 years after the last lower segment Caesarean section, in one case spreading anterolaterally to involve the base of the bladder, and 3 cm of the terminal right ureter, and requiring fairly heroic surgery.

Pathogenesis of adhesions in endometriosis

The presence of peri-endometriotic adhesions and generalized peritoneal adhesions in endometriosis is variable and the coexistence of pelvic inflammatory disease often clouds the operative assessment of adhesions. If spilled blood was the sole aetiological factor in adhesion formation then every woman who spills blood intraperitoneally at ovulation, who experiences retrograde menstruation, or who suffers an intraperitoneal haemorrhage from any cause, should have adhesions.

Microsurgical techniques depend on haemostatic perfection for the excellence of results obtained. However, Nissell & Larsson

(1978) in a study using 120 rats, concluded that it was not the presence of intraperitoneal blood or fibrinogen that caused operative adhesions, but rather surgical trauma, presumably with prostaglandin release.

In order to clarify the pathogenesis of adhesions in external endometriosis, Ohtsuka (1980) collected at laparotomy visceral peritoneum with endometriotic lesions and surrounding tissue. Histological changes were studied with scanning and transmission electron microscopy, and fibrinolytic activity was examined by peritoneal and tissue plasminogen activator activity (PAA). His findings show that the peritoneal PAA of endometriosis lesions was decreased compared with normal peritoneum.

Histologically the surface of early endometriosis was covered with peritoneum—one layer of somewhat degenerated mesothelial cells. Normal peritoneum possessed one layer of healthy mesothelial cells with numerous microvilli evenly covering the slightly bulged cell surface. Progression towards the areas of endometriosis and adhesion formation showed degeneration of the surface mesothelium. The surface became swollen and shortened club-shaped microvilli were irregularly distributed over it. These changes worsened nearer the locus of maximum damage where fibrin deposits were observed and the mesothelium was denuded.

Ohtsuka postulated that it was the damage to the mesothelial peritoneal layer and fibrin outpouring that produced adhesions in endometriosis, this process being promoted by decreased fibrinolytic activity in endometriosis lesions.

Pattison et al (1981), however, showed no difference in peritoneal fluid taken from patients with or without laparoscopic evidence of endometriosis in terms of fibrinolytic activity.

Steroid receptors in endometriosis

The role of steroid receptors in the aetiology and maintenance of endometriosis is yet to be precisely determined. Janne et al (1981) believed that endometriosis lesions possess steroid receptors and it is through these specific receptors that the cyclical features of endometriosis lesions occur in relation to the menstrual cycle. Since the clinical response of endometriosis to steroids is used as a form of assessment for therapy, with, for instance, oestrogen, progestins, androgens and Danazol, then the presence or absence of steroid receptors is probably most important not only to the outcome of treatment but also to the natural history of the disease.

Janne et al found, in a study of 41 patients comparing oestrogen receptors and progestogen receptors in normal endometrium with endometriosis lesions, that there were major differences of distribution of cytosol receptors in these different tissue types.

Some 20% of endometriosis specimens lacked receptors, half contained progestin receptors only, and only 30% contained detectable levels of both oestrogen and progestin cytosol receptors. On this basis they classified endometriosis in the three categories:

1. Receptor negative endometriosis
2. Endometriosis containing both oestrogen and progestin receptors
3. Endometriosis containing progestin receptors only.

Their investigations suggested a higher instance of progestin receptors in milder forms of endometriosis so that hormone therapy with progestins is probably most useful in the milder forms of the disease for this reason. Obviously more work needs to be done in this area to lend specificity to hormonal therapeutic regimens in the medical treatment of endometriosis.

Muse and Wilson (1982) summed up the relationship between endometriosis and infertility by proposing a hypothesis that was multivariant and included all or some of the above mechanisms and suggested perhaps all factors have to be individually assessed before appropriate individualized therapy can be determined—a heroic prospect indeed!

REFERENCES

Badawy S Z A, Cuenca V, Stitzel A, Jacobs R D B, Tomar R H 1984 Autoimmune phenomenon in infertile patients with endometriosis. Obstetrics and Gynecology 63:271–275
Bartosic D, Viscarello R R, Damjanov I 1984 Endometriosis as an autoimmune disease. Fertility and Sterility 41:215 (abstract)
Biggs J G S 1981 Polycystic ovary disease: current concepts. Australian and New Zealand Journal of Obstetrics and Gynaecology 21:26–36
Biggs J G S, Thomas F 1981 Sites of steroid production in the polycystic ovary. British Journal of Obstetrics and Gynaecology 88:42–46
Brekken A C, Massey F M 1980 A common adnexal mass in an uncommon patient. Journal of Reproductive Medicine 25:171–172
Brosens I A, Koninckx P R, Corveleyn P A 1978 A study of plasma progesterone, oestradiol-17β, prolactin and LH levels and of the luteal phase appearance of the

ovaries in patients with endometriosis and infertility. British Journal of Obstetrics and Gynaecology 85:246–250

Cheesman K L, Ben-Nun I, Chatterton R, Cohen M R 1982 Relationships of luteinizing hormone, pregnanediol-3 glucuronide and oestriol-16-glucuronide in urine in infertile women with endometriosis. Fertility and Sterility 38:542–544

Chong A, Baggish 1984 Management of pelvic endometriosis by means of intra-abdominal carbon dioxide laser. Fertility and Sterility 41:14–19

Coulam C B, Hill L M, Breckle R 1982 Ultrasonic evidence for luteinization of unruptured preovulatory follicles. Fertility and Sterility 37:524–529

Cullen T S 1896 Adenomyoma of the round ligament. Bulletin of the Johns Hopkins Hospital 7:112–113

Devroey P, Temmorman M, Verhoevin N et al 1983 Recurrence of the luteinized unruptured follicle. British Journal of Obstetrics and Gynaecology 90:381–382

Dewhurst J 1981 Integrated obstetrics and gynaecology for post graduates. 3rd ed. Blackwell Scientific, Oxford, Ch 32, p 536

Dizerega G S, Barber D C, Hodgen G D 1980 Endometriosis: role of ovarian steroids in initiation, maintenance and suppression. Fertility and Sterility 33:649–653

Dmowski W P, Rao R, Scommegna A 1980 The luteinized unruptured follicle syndrome and endometriosis. Fertility and Sterility 33:30–34

Dmowski W P, Steele R W, Baker G F 1981 Deficient cellular immunity in endometriosis. American Journal of Obstetrics and Gynecology 141:377–388

Donnez J, Langerrock S, Thomas K 1983 Peritoneal fluid volume, 17β oestradiol and progesterone concentrations, in women with endometriosis and or luteinized unruptured follicle syndrome. Gynecologic and Obstetric Investigation 16:210–220

Drake T S, Metz S A, Grunert G M, O'Brien W F 1980 Peritoneal fluid volume in endometriosis. Fertility and Sterility 34:280–281

Drake T S, O'Brien W F, Ramwell P W, Metz S A 1981 Peritoneal fluid thromboxane B2 and 6 keto-prostaglandin F1α in endometriosis. American Journal of Obstetrics and Gynecology 140:401–404

El Mahgoub S, Yaseen S 1980 A positive proof of the theory of coelomic metaplasia. American Journal of Obstetrics and Gynecology 137:137–140

Elstein M, Filho C I 1980 Endometriosis—continuing conundrum. British Medical Journal 281:1427

Gibbons W E, Buttram V C, Rossavik I K 1984 Observed incidence of luteinized unruptured follicles in a population of infertile women undergoing ovulation monitoring by ultrasound. Fertility and Sterility 41:19S (abstract)

Gjönnaess H 1984 Polycystic ovarian syndrome treated by ovarian electrocautery through the laparoscope. Fertility and Sterility 41:20–25

Halban J 1924 Hysteroadenosis metastatick. Wien Klin Wchnschr 37:1205

Halme J, Becker S, Hammond M G, Raj M H, Raj S 1983 Increased activation of pelvic macrophages in infertile women with mild endometriosis. American Journal of Obstetrics and Gynecology 145:333–337

Hambrick I S, Abcarian H, Smith D 1979 Perineal endometriosis in episiotomy incisions: clinical features and management. Diseases of Colon and Rectum 22:550–552

Hirschowitz J S, Soler N G, Worstman J 1978 The galactorrhoea–endometriosis syndrome. Lancet 1:896–898

Hjortrup A, Kehlet H, Lockwood K, Hasiver E 1983 Long-term clinical effects of ovarian wedge resection in polycystic ovary syndrome. Acta Obstetrica et Gynaecologica Scandinavica 62:55–57

Iwanhoff N S 1898 Monattscarift für Geburtschilfe und Gynäkologie 7:195

Jänne O, Kaupilla A, Kokko E, Lantto T, Rönnberg L, Vikho R 1981 Estrogen and progestin receptors in endometriosis lesions: comparisons with endometrial tissue. American Journal of Obstetrics and Gynecology 145:562–566

41

Endometriosis

Javert C T 1951 Observations on the pathology and spread of endometriosis based on the theory of benign metastasis. American Journal of Obstetrics and Gynecology 62:477–481

Jewelewicz R 1975 Management of infertility resulting from anovulation. American Journal of Obstetrics and Gynecology 122:909–920

Katz M, Carr P J, Cohen B M, Millar R P 1978 Hormonal effects of wedge resection of polycystic ovaries. Obstetrics and Gynecology 51:437–444

Kaunitz A, di Sant'agnese P A 1979 Needle tract endometriosis: an unusual complication of amniocentesis. Obstetrics and Gynecology 546:753–755

Kerin J F, Kirby C, Morris D, McEvoy M, Ward B, Cox L W 1983 Incidence of the luteinized unruptured follicle phenomenon in cycling women. Fertility and Sterility 46:620–626

Koninckx P R, Heyns W J, Coruezeyn P R, Brosens I A 1978 Delayed onset of luteinization as a cause of infertility. Fertility and Sterility 29:266–269

Koninckx P R, DeMoor P, Brosens I A 1980a Diagnosis of the luteinized unruptured follicle syndrome by steroid hormone assays of peritoneal fluid. British Journal of Obstetrics and Gynaecology 87:929–934

Koninckx P R, Ide P, Van Den Brocke W, Brosens I A 1980b New aspects of the pathophysiology of endometriosis and associated infertility. Journal of Reproductive Medicine 24:257–260

Koninckx P R, Brosens I A 1982 The luteinized unruptured follicle syndrome In: Wynn R M (ed) Obstetrics and gynaecology annual Vol. 2. Appleton Centenary Crofts, Chicago, p 175–186

Liukkonen S, Koskimies A I, Tenhunen A, Ylostalo P 1984 Diagnosis of luteinized unruptured follicle (LUF) syndrome by ultrasound. Fertility and Sterility 41:26–30

McVeigh J S 1955 An origin of endometriosis theory based on histological morphology. New Zealand Medical Journal 54:346–349

Marik J, Hulka J 1978 Luteinized unruptured follicle syndrome: a subtle cause of infertility. Fertility and Sterility 29:270–274

Meyer R 1903 Ueber eine adenomatose. Wucherung der serosa in einer Bauchnabe. Zeitschrift fur Geburtshilfe und Gynakologie 49:32–45

Moon Y S, Leung P C S, Yuen B H, Gomel V 1981 Prostaglandin F in human endometriotic tissue. American Journal of Obstetrics and Gynecology 141:344–345

Muscato J J, Hamey A F, Weinberg J B 1982 Sperm phagocytosis by human peritoneal macrophages: a possible cause of infertility in endometriosis. American Journal of Obstetrics and Gynecology 144:503–510

Muse K, Wilson E A 1982 How does mild endometriosis cause infertility? Fertility and Sterility 38:145–152

Muse K, Wilson E A, Jawad M J 1982 Prolactin hyperstimulation in response to thyrotropin-releasing hormone in patients with endometriosis. Fertility and Sterility 38:419–422

Navrital E, Kramer A 1936 Endometriose in der Armmuskulatur. Klin Wchnschr 15:1765–1770

Nisell H, Larsson B 1978 Role of blood and fibrinogen in development of intraperitoneal adhesions in rats. Fertility and Sterility 30:470–473

Ohtsuka N 1980 Study of pathogenesis of adhesions in endometriosis. Acta Obstetrica et Gynaecologica Japonica 32:1758–1766

Olive D L, Franklin R R, Gratkins L V 1982 The association between endometriosis and spontaneous abortion: a retrospective study. Journal of Reproductive Medicine 27:333–338

Pattison H A, Koninckx P R, Brosens I A, Vermylen J 1981 Clotting and fibrinolytic activities in peritoneal fluid. British Journal of Obstetrics and Gynaecology 88:160–166

Pick L 1905 Ueber Adenome der mannlichen und weiblichen keimdruse bei

Hermaphroditismus verus und spurius; nebst Bemerkungen uber das endometrium ahnlicke Adenom am inneren weiblicher Genitale. Berl Klin Wchnschr XLII:502–509

Rock J A, Dubin M H, Ghodgankor R B, Berquist C A, Erozan Y S, Kimball A W 1982 Cul de sac fluid in women with endometriosis: fluid volume and prostanoid concentration during the proliferative phase of the cycle—days 8 to 12. Fertility and Sterility 37:747–752

Sampson J A 1922 The life history of ovarian haematomas (haemorrhagic cysts) of endometrial (Müllerian) type. American Journal of Obstetrics and Gynecology 4:451–456

Stein I F, Leventhal M L 1935 Amenorrhoea associated with bilateral polycystic ovaries. American Journal of Obstetrics & Gynecology 29:181–191

TeLinde R W, Scott R B 1951 External endometriosis. Clinical and experimental. American Surgeon 17:397–405

Vaitukaitis J C 1983 Polycystic ovary syndrome—what is it? New England Journal of Medicine 309:1245–1246

Von Recklinghausen F 1885 Veber die venose embolic und den regrograden transport in den venen und in den lymphgefassen. Virchows Archives (Pathology: Anatomy) 100:503

Weed J C 1980 Prostaglandins as related to endometriosis. Clinical Obstetrics and Gynaecology 23:894–901

Weed J C, Arquembourg 1980 Endometriosis: can it produce an autoimmune response resulting in infertility? Clinical Obstetrics and Gynaecology 23:885–893

Ylikorkala O, Tenhunen A 1984 Follicular fluid prostaglandins in endometriosis and ovarian hyperstimulation. Fertility and Sterility 41:66–69

Zumoff B, Freeman R, Coupey S, Saenger P, Markowitz M, Kream J 1983 A chronobiologic abnormality in LH secretion in teenage girls with the polycystic ovary syndrome. New England Journal of Medicine 309:1206–1209

4

Pathology and staging of endometriosis

Gross pathology

The age, location and extent or stage of individual lesions of endometriosis determines the gross pathological picture.

The earliest recognizable and histologically proven gross lesions are seen macroscopically as blister-like vesicles, 2–3 mm in diameter, on the surface of target organs or peritoneum, containing clear fluid and showing no evidence of haemorrhage. On microscopic section, these lesions show a typical endometrial glandular appearance with clear fluid filled 'cysts'. This is the stage before haemorrhage into these lesions occurs and before the classic powder burn—chocolate cyst appearance that has, in the past, been commonly described as 'typical early endometriosis'.

In the Brisbane series two-thirds of the 53 patients demonstrating this earliest recognizable stage of the disease also had concurrently, more extensive stages of the disease and in only 18 cases was it the sole diagnostic stigma of endometriosis.

These lesions have been called stage 0 lesions in the Brisbane series; occult endometriosis is another description for these lesions.

Endometriosis seldom occurs as a solitary lesion but when it does it can still exhibit the total gambit of destructive activity. It is also a disease that seldom affects extragenital organs without pelvic involvement. In the Brisbane series there were four such patients with endometriosis involving the small bowel (1 case) which is exceptionally rare, appendix (1 case) and large bowel (2 cases) and no involvement macroscopically of uterus, adnexa, or pelvic peritoneum. The true incidence, of course, of intra-abdominal endometriosis is totally unknown since only those cases operated on have been diagnosed in the Brisbane series.

Location of disease

The locations of endometriosis in 717 patients in the Brisbane series are shown in Table 4.1. Obviously there are no cases in this series of remote extra-pelvic lesions although the author has seen cases involving umbilicus, breast, and inguinal lymph glands being treated elsewhere in Brisbane during the time of this study.

Table 4.1 Location of endometriosis

1. Pouch of Douglas	502	
2. Utero-sacral ligaments	278	
3. Pelvic peritoneum	254	
4. Left ovary	245	} both ovaries 58
5. Right ovary	242	
6. Bladder	108	
7. Uterine surface	67	
8. Rectovaginal septum	47	
9. Right tube	43	} both tubes 7
10. Left tube	41	
11. Bowel	40	
12. Appendix	38	
13. Vagina	9	
14. Cervix	2	
15. Wound	2	
16. Ureter	2	

These locations recorded are quite different to those of Mettler (1982) and Blaustein (1982). Mackay et al (1983) quoted a collected series of over 1000 cases where the disease was confined to the ovary, pelvic peritoneum of the pouch of Douglas and the utero-sacral ligaments in most cases, a similar picture to that of the Brisbane series. The gross pathological picture changes as lesions age, and the repeated cyclical haemorrhage and subsequent red cell breakdown provokes an intense scar tissue reaction cyclically, until the endometrioma often becomes totally buried in scar tissue, which on section shows a central chocolate area perhaps only equal to 10% or less of the diameter of the lesion. The fact that such lesions encased in dense scar tissue are still perfused cyclically with hormones which stimulate the haemorrhagic response at menstruation, often leaves one agog. Of course, the vascular perfusion does, on occasion, become inadequate because of scar tissue, leading to avascular necrosis.

Microscopic appearance

The gross lesions on microscopy may fail to show the classic appearance of extrauterine endometrial glandular tissue because the glandular tissue has been either destroyed by avascular necrosis, consequent on the incremental compression effect of cyclical encysted haemorrhage, altered by squamous metaplasia, or been destroyed as a result of the overall destructive nature of the disease itself.

The surrounding thickened tissues around endometriomata usually demonstrate macrophages laden with blood pigment interspersed in a fibroblastic stroma, and even though there may not be recognizable endometrial tissue, it is still identifiable as endometriosis (Blaustein 1982).

A great variability of appearance can exist in one section depending on the age of the lesion. Sometimes when only stroma predominates, the term 'stromal endometriosis' may be used as a descriptive subclassification of endometriosis.

Endosalpingiosis

This condition was found three times in the Brisbane series and is characterized by endometriosis-like cysts lined with epithelium resembling endosalpinx. The histogenesis of this type of lesion is undoubtedly by metaplasia. Ernst et al (1981) carried out a study in infertile women with this disease and noted that it was associated with tubal diverticulum formation, thickening of the muscularis layer of the tube, and with altered tubal physiology and infertility. Tutschka & Lauchlan (1980), on the other hand, considered endosalpingiosis to be homologous with endometriosis and of no serious prognostic association. This was certainly the Brisbane experience as all three cases were multiparous and the histological diagnosis was felt to be of academic interest only.

Endosalpingiosis shares the same relationship via à vis the serous tumours, as does endometriosis to endometrial tumours. The histological picture, which is the way in which endosalpingiosis is histologically distinguished from stage 0 endometriosis lesions (Fig. 4.1), usually consists of one layer of well demarcated columnar or cuboidal cells, with ciliated cells and pale secretory cells, usually with peg cells (Fig. 4.2). There is often an association with psammoma bodies (Fig. 4.3) which is not a feature of uncomplicated endometriosis. Unlike endometriosis, the stroma shows none of the loose vascularized characteristics of endometrial stroma.

Endosalpingiosis may rarely be associated with 'endocervicosis' where ectopically located endocervical epithelium occurs. These

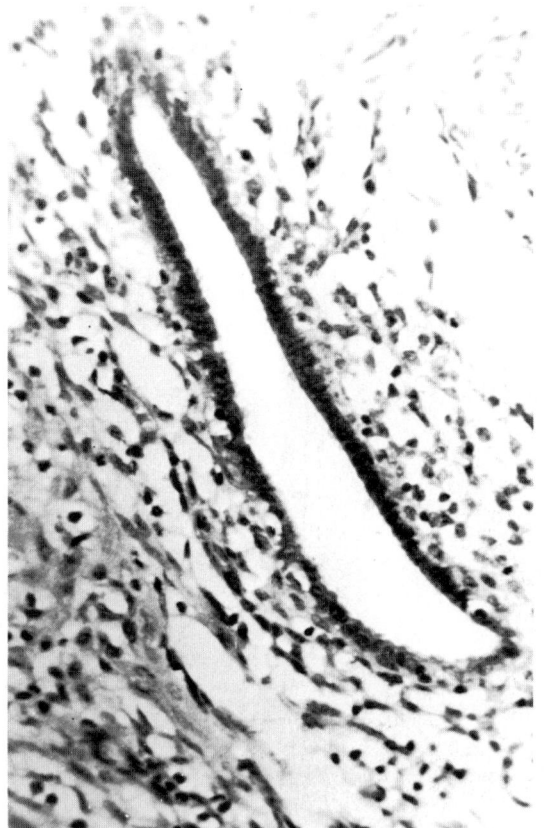

Fig. 4.1 Stage 0 endometriosis with no evidence of haemorrhage

lesions are all derivatives of coelomic epithelium which has its origins in mesoderm, so perhaps they ought to be more properly called mesotheliomas. As Tutschka & Lauchlan point out this would cause confusion with the well known descriptive word used to describe asbestos-induced tumours. Malignant change in endosalpingiosis if it occurs, is usually either papillary, or serocystadenoma-type cancer.

Endometriosis of the oviduct, occurring in scar tissue after previous tubal surgery, is a separate disease from endosalpingiosis with different histogenesis, morphological appearance and clinical picture (Fig. 4.4). Classically seen after surgical sterilization by tubal diathermy, it can also occur after reconstructive tubal surgery such as reimplantation procedures. Postoperatively the patient develops

47

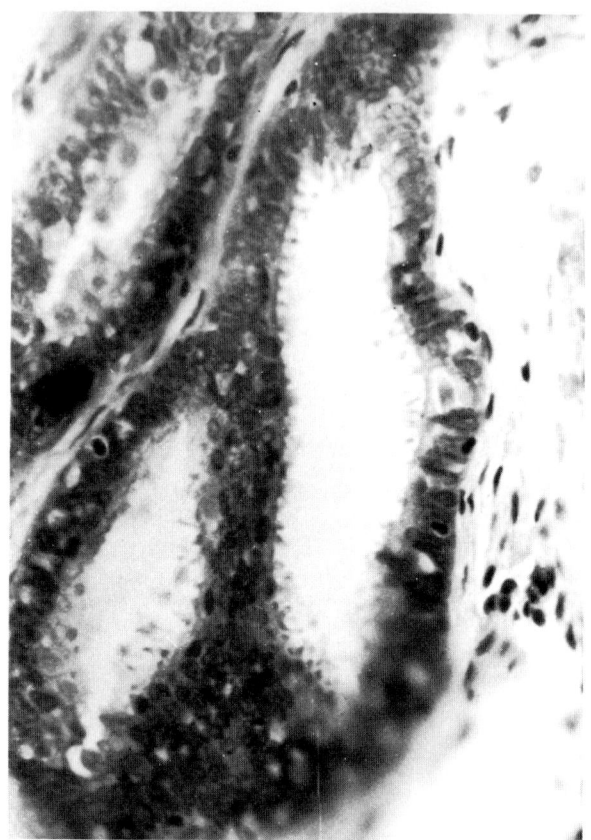

Fig. 4.2 Endosalpingiosis—note cilia and variable cellular lining compared to endometriosis (Fig. 4.1)

a fistula from the uterine cavity through the cornual tubal stump out into the peritoneal cavity. The fistula is lined with endometrium, not endosalpinx, and therefore cyclical bleeding occurs at the site of the fistula producing dysmenorrhoea, dyspareunia, and a tender adnexal swelling, all of which are localized to the site of the tubal endometrioma.

This condition was recognized in five patients in the Brisbane series, three of whom had previously undergone bilateral, unipolar tubal diathermy for sterilization. The other two patients had had tubal reimplantations and one of these had an ectopic pregnancy at one tubal reimplantation site which was disrupted, and an endometrioma at the other contralateral site of reanastomosis.

According to Dewhurst (1981) this condition is usually found in

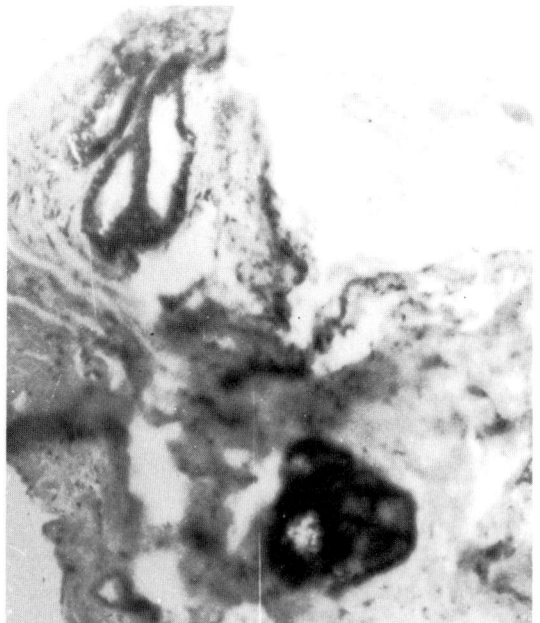

Fig. 4.3 Histological section of endosalpingiosis showing psammoma body

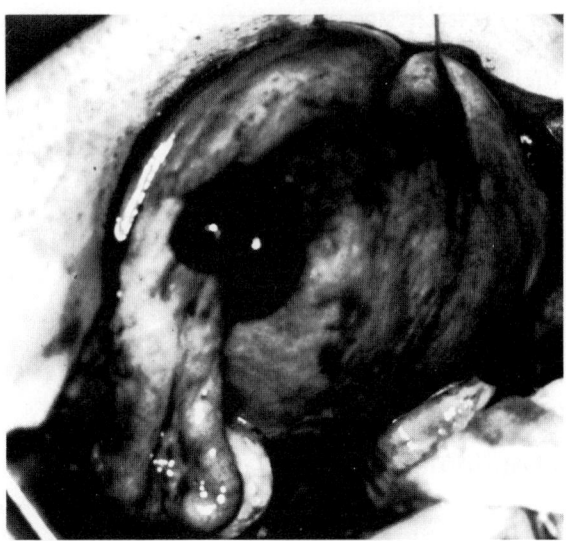

Fig. 4.4 Operative photograph showing a dramatic tubal endometrioma after previous tubal sterilization by electrodiathermy (courtesy of Dr L Brunello)

multiparous patients and it is thought that repeated pregnancies and repeated vigorous curettage might predispose to the endometrium extending into the myometrium.

In the Brisbane series 59 of 717 patients had coexistent adenomyosis, and this would not seem to be a significant coexistence since a further 146 patients during this time were histologically diagnosed as having significant adenomyosis without endometriosis. Dewhurst quoted a coincidence of 10–20% between the two conditions. Moreover, they can coincidentally both coexist with other evidence of luteal inadequacies such as polycystic ovary disease, endometrial hyperplasia, and benign mammary dysplasia. The ease with which some histologists find adenomyosis in hysterectomy specimens has been noted by Joel-Cohen (1978), but it is better to rely on histological confirmation of a clinical diagnosis to achieve a satisfactory incidence. In adenomyosis, the multiple, usually symmetrically disposed, intramural uterine lesions lead to a tender enlargement of the uterus which, on direct visualization, shows a characteristic gentle diffuse undulating surface irregularity. On sectioning of the uterus, this is shown to be due to collections of small pale fibrous areas in the myometrium with some central haemorrhagic areas. Clinically the disease produces symptoms of endometriosis (dysmenorrhoea, dyspareunia, menorrhagia) and the signs of fibroids (uterine enlargement and tenderness). The simplest form of treatment is a hysterectomy if the patient finds the symptoms intolerable.

Where disseminated adenomyomas of the abdominal and pelvic cavity are found, fortunately a rare condition, the diagnosis will only be made histologically (Bergen et al 1981). It has been suggested such lesions develop from endometrial stromal cells in endometriosis and because these lesions can mimic metastatic cancer, and because of the risk of adenosarcoma occurring in them, extensive surgery followed by (? medical) oophorectomy seems to be the treatment of choice.

Endometriosis in other organ systems

Intestinal endometriosis

Meyer et al (1980) from Germany and Pillay & Hardie (1980) from the Princess Alexandra Hospital, Brisbane writing on intestinal complications of endometriosis, very appropriately remind surgeons of the necessity to consider a diagnosis of endometriosis when confronted with atypical rectal bleeding, pelvic colon strictures, and polypoid colonic masses. The presentation of abdominal endometriosis can be quite varied—Grimes & Fowler (1980) reported a case of caecal adenosquamous carcinoma arising in endometriosis; Honore (1980) described a gut obstruction due to endometriosis in Meckel's diverticulum; Charles & Samyuktha (1979) and Blumenthal (1981) reported cases of umbilical endometriosis while appendiceal endometriosis was discussed by Langman et al (1981). Often in intestinal endometriosis the diagnosis, histologically, might be inconclusive and the possibility of neoplasm has always to be considered.

In the Brisbane series 89 women had their appendix removed during surgery for endometriosis and of these, 39 had histologically proven endometriosis. The histological examination of all 89 excised vermiform appendices revealed a diagnosis of carcinoid tumour in a further two cases and threadworms in two cases.

The incidence of endometriosis involving the bowel (40 cases) is the same as endometriosis involving the appendix in the Brisbane series. This finding is in variance with that reported by Williams & Pratt (1977) who found that in 968 laparotomies 37% of patients with endometriosis had bowel involvement and 9% had appendiceal involvement. Perforation of gastrointestinal endometriosis in pregnancy is rare, although Clement (1977) reported a case of sigmoid colon endometriosis which perforated, and in 1981 Gini et al reported an unfortunate woman who perforated her appendiceal endometrioma at 35 weeks' gestation.

Curiously, the first case of endometriosis seen by the author in his postgraduate career was a 46-year-old gravida 8, para 6 woman who presented with an acute abdomen due to perforated appendiceal endometriosis and who had some 40 discrete lesions on the surface of her large bowel and none involving her uterus, tubes or ovaries— a phenomenon not seen since!

Appendicectomy in endometriosis with infertility

Pittaway (1983) summed up the issue of routine appendicectomy in endometriosis patients as follows:

1. Those endometriosis patients undergoing *non*-infertility surgery should have appendicectomy performed, because there is a significant prevalence of appendiceal endometriosis in endometriosis victims (13%)

2. Those patients having infertility surgery should only have the appendix removed if it is morphologically abnormal. They should not have a normal appendix removed

Pittaway found that in 38% of excised appendices the diagnosis of appendiceal endometriosis was not readily apparent on cursory examination.

Malinak (1980) while acknowledging the controversial nature of endometriosis, infertility, and appendicectomy, and the risk of post-appendicectomy peritonitis further seriously compromising fertility, did not perform routine incidental appendicectomy and confined himself to removal only if, after inspection in every case, there was a suggestion of pathology due to endometriosis, or other processes, involving the appendix.

The author has tended to follow this philosophy which is why some 50% of excised appendices showed significant pathology. The usual gross appearance of the pathologically involved appendix in these patients has been reduction in length, fibrosis of the wall, and a tendency to corkscrew deformity with the appendix assuming a spiral shape. Periappendiceal adhesions are not a noticeable feature of endometriosis of the appendix.

Thoracic endometriosis

Catamenial pneumothorax associated with endometriosis of either pleura or diaphragm, or related to diaphragmatic defects has been described by Yamazaki et al (1980), Furman et al (1980) and Stern et al (1980) who believed catamenial pneumothorax must be endoscopically assessed with a view to surgical closure of diaphragmatic defects if they are of sufficient severity. Standard gynaecological therapy for endometriosis ought to produce long-term cure of the respiratory problem.

In a review of 46 patients with thoracic endometriosis, Hibbard et al (1981) reported that only 17 patients also had proven pelvic endometriosis and they pointed out that in most of the thoracic cases, because there was no coincidental gynaecological evidence of endometriosis, the true pulmonary diagnosis was delayed, prolonging the patients' respiratory disability.

Obviously cyclical symptoms anywhere in the female body should alert medical attendants to the possibility of endometriosis in any organ.

Urinary tract endometriosis

There are many well documented cases of endometriosis of the urinary tract in the literature as well as in the Brisbane series where one in seven affected patients had urinary tract lesions. In fact, Fianu et al (1980) have surgically treated 17 women for bladder endometriosis by excision—including excision of the trigone where indicated—with excellent results and no serious loss of bladder function. Vaginal hysterotomy for legal termination of pregnancy was a common preceding gynaecological event in their patients.

Surgery, according to Denes et al (1980) offered the best therapeutic approach for the rare occurrence of ureteric endometriosis. While Gardner & Whittaker (1981) reported the first case where danazol alone had been used to overcome and reverse endometriosis-induced ureteric obstruction, Pittaway et al (1982) urged caution if using this line of therapy because, in their patient, recurrent obstruction of her ureter by endometriosis occurred within 2 months of the completion of her 9-week course of danazol, 500 mg daily. They make the point that endometriotic ureteric obstruction can be uni- or bilateral and very insidious, as can endometriosis elsewhere, and that silent loss of function can occur in 25% of cases (Moore et al 1979). Initially, Pittaway et al had tried medroxyprogesterone on their patient but this had not helped her symptoms. Gantt et al (1981) documented radiologically the reversal of ureteric obstruction due to surgically proven endometriosis, after progestin therapy.

In the Brisbane series the bladder was affected in 108 cases and the ureter in two—both with extensive involvement. Of the 108 cases of bladder involvement, 97 involved the serosa only, nine the serosa and muscularis and, two the full thickness of the bladder wall, although in neither of these last two patients was there cyclical haematuria or bladder symptoms.

In an interesting case report of intrinsic ureteric obstruction associated with an endometriotic ureteric polyp, Tulusan & Trotnow (1983) posed the question of whether, in their case, the lesion was due to endometriomatous infiltration from without, or was related to an unsuspected ureteric injury at abdominal hysterectomy performed two years previously.

The ureteric involvement cases in the Brisbane series both followed previous lower segment Caesarean section and in both cases the lower course of the involved ureters were shown to be embedded in endometriotic scar tissue. The aid of a specialist urology surgeon colleague was enlisted to reconstruct urinary conduit continuity after resection of endometriomatous tissue. One difficulty in bladder resection is to know when resection is clear of endometriotic infiltration of the bladder wall.

Malignant tumours in endometriosis

The association between endometriosis and malignant change was initially noted by Sampson (1925). The frequency with which endometriosis undergoes malignant change is unkown. Mostoufiza-deh & Scully (1980) state the incidence of coincident endometriosis in known ovarian malignancy has been recorded as a range of 11–28% of cases while endometrioid cancer originating directly from ovarian tissue has been recorded as 1–24% in various series.

There are two main groups of cancer arising from endometriosis—mainly endometrioid tumours that histologically resemble any malignant tumour arising in endometrium; and common epithelial-type tumours including clear cell cancer, and the rarer serous, muscinous and squamous cell cancers.

Endometrioid cancer

The age incidence of endometrioid cancer in patients with endometriosis was demonstrated to be around a decade younger than in patients with endometrioid cancer in general. Aure et al (1971) found 26% of patients with ovarian cancer and endometriosis were less than 40 years of age at diagnosis compared with 8% where there was no endometriosis. Fathalla (1967) found that pain was the commonest symptom and was most likely caused by bleeding from the endometriosis rather than from the tumour. She believed the diagnostic clue to malignant change was when the pain altered from its usual periodic pattern to a constant pain. Since rupture of benign endometriotic cysts is rare—a fact corroborated by the Brisbane series—she believed that evidence of rupture was highly suggestive of malignant change.

The most common gross expression of cancer arising in an endometrioma is a papillary or polypoid mass on the cut surface, or an exceptionally large endometrioma of more than 15 cm diameter.

Histologically pure adenocarcinomas and adenocanthomas of endometrioid type occur with equal frequency. Generally speaking premalignant endometrial changes such as adenomatous or atypical hyperplasia should also be encountered in endometriosis and it seems reasonable to assume such lesions have the same malignant potential as in the endometrium.

Clear cell cancer

There is stronger circumstantial evidence for the origin of endometriosis in some clear cell ovarian cancers. Russell (1979) found a 49% frequency of biopsy proven endometriosis in 33 cases of clear cell ovarian cancer with only a 28% frequency in 72 cases of endometrioid cancer, while Scully et al (1966) showed 25% of both endometrioid and clear cell cancers arose in endometriosis. The association between this form of cancer, believed to be of mesonephric origin, and endometriosis is unclear. While occasionally these tumours are solid in the wall of an endometriotic cyst, they are more often single or multiple papillary masses inside an endometriotic cyst.

Other epithelial cancers

Russell (1979) found that only 3% of 233 cases of ovarian serous cancer, and 4% of 69 cases of ovarian muscinous cancer had endometriosis. This low coincidence figure is probably related to the fact that such cancers rarely arise in endometrial tissues.

However, the only case of coincidental ovarian cancer found in the 717 cases of the Brisbane series had both stage III endometriosis and stage III papillary serous ovarian cancer. She is alive and well 3 years after radical surgery and chemotherapy and apparently free of both disease processes.

Endometrial sarcomas

Stromal sarcomas, malignant mixed mesodermal tumours, and mesodermal adenosarcomas have all been described arising in endometrium and are rare in endometriosis. Crum et al (1981) reported a sad, fascinating case of a patient previously reported because of extensive polypoid abdominal endometriosis, who was treated by radiotherapy to obliterate ovarian function because she refused medical therapy, and in whom there subsequently developed a fatal sarcomatous change in the irradiated endometriosis.

Cancers arising in extra-ovarian endometriosis

According to Brooks & Wheeler (1977) almost one-quarter of cases of malignancy in endometriosis occur in non-ovarian locations.

Endometrioid cancer

Mostoufizadeh & Scully (1980) were aware of 35 cases of endometrioid cancer reportedly arising in non-ovarian endometriosis. The age range was 30–73 years with an average of 48. Two-thirds of the patients were nulliparous and two had previously been on long-term oestrogen therapy, two had prior resection of ovarian endometriosis showing atypical endometrial hyperplasia, and two had coincident oestrogen-secreting ovarian tumours.

Thirteen of these non-ovarian tumours were in the recto-vaginal septum, four in the vagina, three in the bladder and others involved the fallopian tube, uterine cervix, corpus and utero-sacral ligaments, large and small bowel, and umbilicus as well as a questionable lymph node cancer.

Twenty-eight of the tumours were adenocarcinomas and seven were adenoacanthomas.

As a result of histological, histochemical and ultrastructure studies, Stenback and Kauppila (1981) concluded that endometroid ovarian adenocarcinoma consisted of two types of structure: one was also found in endometriosis and was similar to endometrium, while the other had a surface ultrastructure more consistent with Mullerian derived coelomic origin.

Non-carcinomatous tumour of non-ovarian origin

Berkowitz et al (1978) reported on vaginal endometriosis producing endometrial stromal sarcoma and 14 cases of endometrioid stromal sarcoma occurring in women from 20 to 64 years of age were located in the recto-vaginal septum, large bowel, bladder, vagina, tube, omentum and pleura. The survival rate after therapy does not seem to relate to the degree of malignancy of the tumour or its location.

Endometriotic polyposis

Polypoid endometriosis is rare and the Greek woman previously reported from New York as dying from sarcoma after radiotherapy (Crum et al 1981) was such a case.

Malignant transformation of endometriosis

Clearly almost any type of malignancy can develop in endometriosis and since conclusively documented cases of malignant transformation are rare, the incidence is unknown. In the Brisbane series it was exceedingly rare, which may be related to the low incidence of such malignancy in the community, or the high incidence of early active treatment of early stage endometriosis in the Brisbane series, or to other unrecognized factors.

For completeness in this review of endometrioid cancer arising in locations other than the female uterus, mention is made of three cases of endometrioid cancer of the prostate in three males receiving oestrogen therapy presented to a meeting of the Royal Society of Medicine by Jurewicz et al (1983). The histological findings of endometrial cancer of the prostate suggested a possible origin in endometrial glandules of mullerian origin persisting in the uterus masculinis and possible remaining oestrogen sensitive. Radiotherapy was successfully used in these cases.

Classification—staging of endometriosis

There is a great need for a universally accepted classification or staging system for endometriosis if results of treatment from different centres around the world, using different therapeutic modalities, are to be meaningful and truly comparable.

Acosta et al (1973) acknowledged that there was at that time no useful means by which a reasonable prognosis can be offered to an infertile patient following conservative surgery for endometriosis. They drew up a classification (Table 4.2) based on a study of 107 such infertile patients so treated which they hoped would establish predictions for future conceptions. The results of treatment in these patients showed that the duration of infertility was significant in terms of fertility outcome—the pregnancy rate decreased with the length of infertility. Another variable in predicting results was patient age at time of operation—the success rate fell from 52% in the under 25 age group to 25% in the over 35 years group. Acosta et al found that the correlation between pregnancy rate and degree of endometriosis was 75% success in mild, 50% in moderate and 33% in severe cases.

Kistner et al (1977) presented a suggested classification for endometriosis (Table 4.3). In addition to the factors considered by

Table 4.2 Acosta classification

Classification	Description
Mild	1. Scattered lesions in the anterior or posterior cul-de-sac or pelvic peritoneum (no scarring) 2. Rare surface implant on ovarian surface with no scarring or adhesions 3. No peritubular adhesions
Moderate	1. Involvement of one or both ovaries with several surface lesions and scarring retraction and endometrioma formation with associated 2. Minimal periovarian and minimal peritubular adhesions 3. Superificial implants in anterior and posterior cul-de-sac with scarring and retraction but not sigmoid invasion
Severe	1. Endometriosis involving one or both ovaries with endometriomata $> 2 \times 2$ cm 2. One or both ovaries bound down by adhesions associated with endometriosis with or without tubal adhesions to ovaries 3. One or both tubes bound down or obstructed by endometriosis; associated adhesions or lesions 4. Obliteration of the cul-de-sac from adhesions or lesions associated with endometriosis 5. Thickening of the uterosacral ligaments and cul-de-sac lesions from invasive endometriosis with obliterations of the cul-de-sac 6. Bowel or urinary tract involvement

Acosta et al, they noted that previous pelvic surgery for endometriosis, with the presence of peritubal adhesions and endosalpinx damage, diminished the possibility of pregnancy, and that while 35% of patients were pregnant within 1 year of surgery, a further 15–20% became pregnant by the second year. They reported luteal phase insufficiency in 25% of patients having surgery for ovarian endometriosis and believed that this factor, if untreated, could contribute to delay in conception. More recently Pittaway et al (1983) did not detect luteal phase defects in patients with endometriosis, so postoperative occurrences may have been related to the surgery rather than to the disease.

In an effort to equate results with the extent of the endometriosis a very detailed classification, with illustrations, was provided which was based largely on the natural history of the disease, as far as it is known.

This classification suffers from the fact that non-genital endometriosis only comes in at stage IV, when in fact involvement in the Brisbane series was common at Kistner stage I in many cases of bladder endometriosis and some cases of bowel and appendiceal endometriosis.

Buttram (1978) proposed expansions of existing systems but he

Table 4.3 Kistner classification

Classification	Description
Stage I	Broad ligaments: no implants > 5 mm Tubes: avascular adhesions, fimbria free Ovaries: avascular adhesions, no fixation Cul-de-sac: no implants > 5 mm Bowel and appendix: normal
Stage IIA	Broad ligaments: no implants > 5 mm Tubes: avascular adhesions, fimbria free Ovaries: endometrial cyst 5 cm or less—A1 stage 　　　　　endometrial cyst > 5 cm—A2 stage 　　　　　endometrial cyst ruptured—A3 stage Cul-de-sac: no implants > 5 mm Bowel and appendix: normal
Stage IIB	Broad ligaments: covered by adherent ovary Tubes: adhesions not removable by endoscopy, fimbria free Ovaries: fixed to the broad ligament, implants > 5 m Cul-de-sac: multiple implants, no adherent bowel or fixed uterus Bowel and appendix: normal
Stage III	Broad ligaments: may be covered by adherent tube or ovary Tubes: fimbria are covered by adhesions Ovaries: adherent with or without implants or endometriomata Cul-de-sac: multiple implants, no adherent bowel or fixed uterus Bowel, appendix and bladder: normal
Stage IV	Bladder: implants Uterus: may be fixed and adherent posteriorly Cul-de-sac: covered by adherent bowel or fixed retrodisplaced uterus Bowel: adherent to the cul-de-sac, uterosacral ligaments, or corpus Appendix: may be involved

proposed using up to 10 descriptive allocations per patient and this seemed to be unduly complicated. In December 1979, the American Fertility Society (AFS) produced a classification based on a point score system (Table 4.4) and drawn up by a committee of experts in the field of endometriosis—Andrews, Behrman, Buttram, Cohen, Eward, Jones, Kistner, Thomas and Weed.

The Society produced a standard sheet for gynaecologists to complete which included a small diagram for representing the location. The diagram is similar to that used in the Brisbane series. Hassan (1981) noted that the AFS classification did not emphasize disease of the utero-sacral ligaments which he considered important, and he believed a three-dimensional volumetric assessment of endometriotic lesions was more representative than two-dimensional surface representation. Andrews (1981) noted the continuing need for a system of classification that satisfied all comparison require-

Endometriosis

Table 4.4 American Fertility Society classification

Stage I	(mild)	1–5 points
Stage II	(moderate)	6–15 points
Stage III	(severe)	16–30 points
Stage IV	(extensive)	31–54 points

Peritoneum

Endometriosis	<1 cm	1–3 cm	>3 cm
	1	2	3
Adhesions	Filmy	Dense + partial obliteration of cul-de-sac	Dense + complete obliteration of cul-de-sac
	1	2	3

Ovary

Endometriosis	<1 cm	1–3 cm	>3 cm or ruptured endometrioma
R	2	4	6
L	2	4	6
Adhesions	Filmy	Dense + partial ovarian enclosure	Dense + complete ovarian enclosure
R	2	4	6
L	2	4	6

Tube

Endometriosis	<1 cm	>1 cm	Tubal occlusion
R	2	4	6
L	2	4	6
Adhesions	Filmy	Dense + tubal distortion	Dense + tubal enclosure
R	2	4	6
L	2	4	6

ments. He also noted that while some workers believed the size of the lesions was important, he, like Dmowski (1980), believed bilaterality was also very important in the prognosis for fertility.

Two hundred and fourteen women with endometriosis treated at Johns Hopkins Hospital, Baltimore, from 1960 to 1979 were reviewed by Rock et al (1981). These patients were treated by conservative surgery alone and 115 (54%) conceived following surgery, of whom 109 produced a live child. They also found a reduction in the spontaneous abortion rate from 49% to 20% after conservative surgery for secondary infertility. However, they found that for the American Fertility Society Classification to reveal significant differences in fecundability, categories have to be combined, for example 'mild + moderate' versus 'severe + extensive'. They also found that where ovarian endometriomata greater than 3 cm existed or had ruptured, there was a significant reduction in pregnancy success rate.

In 1982 Guzick et al recommended that the American Fertility Society classification be modified so that the arbitrary individual

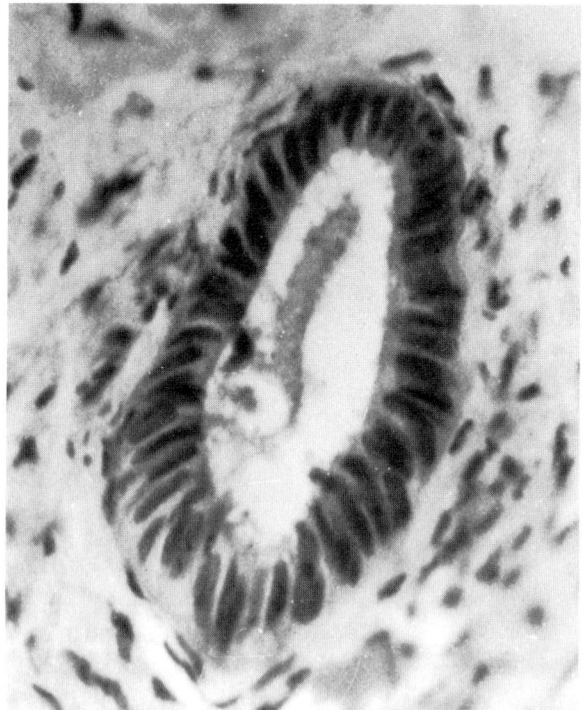

Fig. 4.5 Endometriosis stage 0

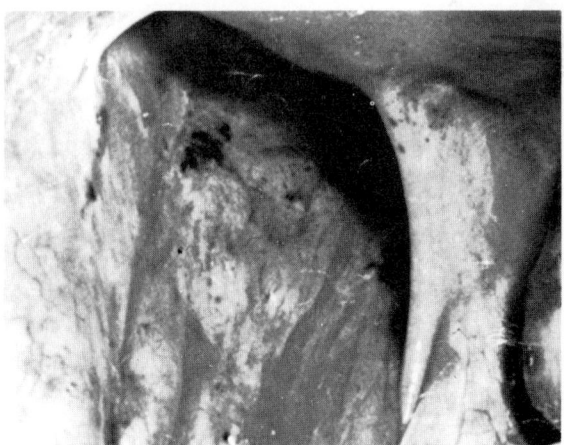

Fig. 4.6 Endometriosis stage I. Lesions in pouch of Douglas and on left utero-sacral ligament

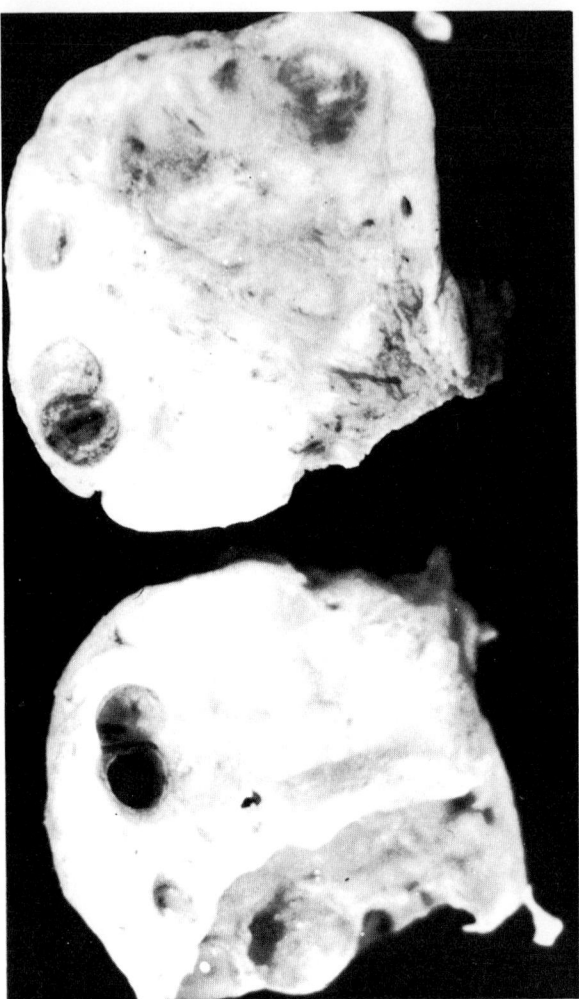

Fig. 4.7 Endometriosis stage II

category point scores or weights were replaced with empirically derived weights as they felt the AFS scale specified poorly the relationship between severity of disease and post-therapy pregnancy success rate because of the arbitrary point score 'cut offs'. Later, in 1982, Adamson et al showed that neither the Acosta nor the Kistner classifications, in their study of 123 women, predicted pregnancy outcome. They believed 'clustering' techniques would be useful in determining new combinations of variables when attempting to forecast pregnancy outcome.

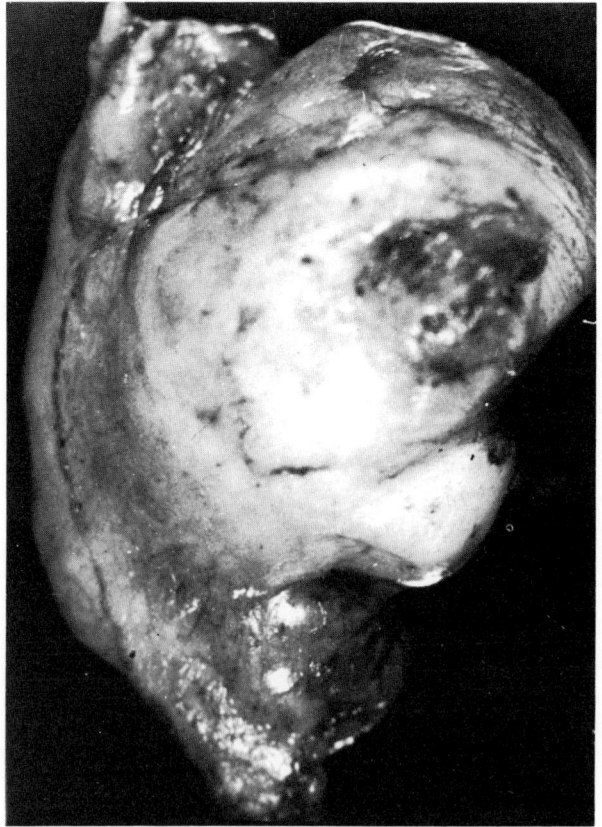

Fig. 4.8 Endometriosis stage III. Destructive disease in a polycystic ovary—unopened

The simple classification used in the Brisbane series (Table 4.5) (Figs. 4.5–4.9) is based on severity and extent of disease, irrespective of organ involved and the staging follows what was perceived years ago to be a simple natural history of the disease.

Table 4.5 The Brisbane series classification

Stage	Extent of disease	No.
Stage 0	Minimal disease + no haemorrhage	18
Stage I	Minimal disease + haemorrhage + no adhesions	241
Stage II	Progression with haemorrhage + adhesions	254
Stage III	Progression to organ destruction + dense adhesions	165
Stage IV	Total loss of reproductive function + extensive organ destruction: dense adhesions progressed to 'frozen pelvis'	39

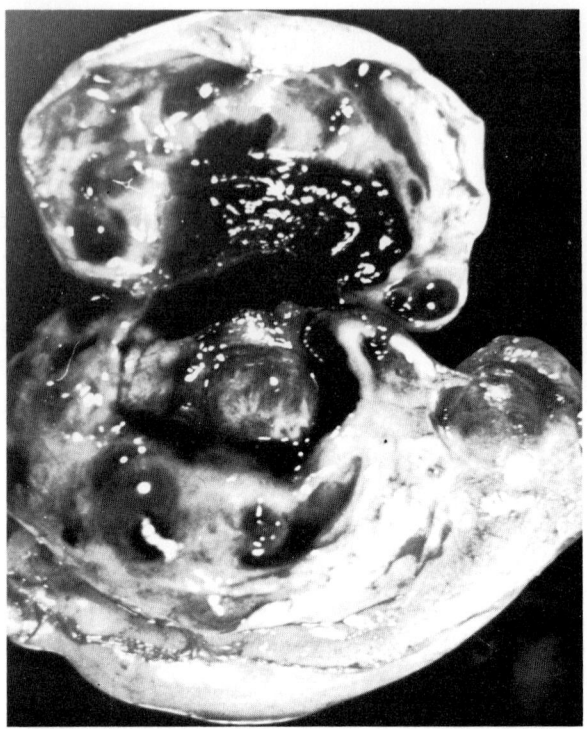

Fig. 4.9 Endometriosis stage III. Destructive disease in a polycystic ovary—opened

Until something more appropriate is produced, there is no proposal to abandon it. The question of bilaterality mentioned previously is perhaps important although a revision of Table 4.1 shows bilateral disease involvement is not all that common and it is possible that a unilateral stage III ovarian lesion is of greater prognostic significance than bilateral stage I ovarian lesions. It is believed that progressive damage and loss of organ function is as important as bilaterality, especially if one accepts that prostaglandin levels in peritoneal fluid in the infertile patients with endometriosis rise as the degree and extent of damage to tissue increases, with greater impedence of fertility factors.

REFERENCES

Acosta A A, Buttram V C Jr, Besch P K, Malinak L R, Franklin R R, Vanderheyden J D 1973 A proposed classification of endometriosis. Obstetrics and Gynecology 42:19–25

Adamson G D, Frison L, Lamb E J 1982 Endometriosis: studies for a method for the design of a surgical staging system. Fertility and Sterility 38:659–666

American Fertility Society 1979 Classification of endometriosis. Fertility and Sterility 32:633–634

Andrews W C 1981 Classification of endometriosis. Fertility and Sterility 35:124–125

Aure J C, Heg K, Kolstad P 1971 Carcinoma of the ovary and endometriosis. Acta Obstetrica et Gynecologica Scandinavica 50:63–67

Bergen S, Owen J, Snider W R, Lim Y C 1981 Disseminated adenomyomas of the abdominal and pelvic cavities: a case report. American Surgeon 47:232–235

Berkowitz R S, Ehrmann R L, Knapp R C 1978 Endometrial stromal sarcoma arising from vaginal endometriosis. Obstetrics and Gynecology 51 (Suppl 2):345–375

Blaustein A 1982 Pathology of the female genital tract, 2nd edn. Springer Verlag, New York, p 464–478

Blumenthal N J 1981 Umbilical endometriosis: a case report. South African Medical Journal 59:198–199

Brooks J, Wheeler J 1977 Malignancy arising in extragonadal endometriosis. Cancer 40:3065–3073

Buttram V C Jr 1978 An expanded classification of endometriosis. Fertility and Sterility 30:240–242

Charles S X, Samyuktha K 1979 Endometriosis of umbilicus. Australian and New Zealand Journal of Obstetrics and Gynaecology 19:239–240

Clement P 1977 Perforation of the sigmoid colon during pregnancy—a rare complication of endometriosis. British Journal of Obstetrics and Gynaecology 84:548–550

Crum C P, Wible J, Frick H C, Fenolico C M, Richart R M, Williamson S 1981 A case of extensive pelvic endometriosis terminating in endometrial sarcoma. American Journal of Obstetrics and Gynecology 140:718–719

Denes F T, Pompio A C, Montelatto N, Lopes R 1980 Ureteral endometriosis. International Urology and Nephrology 12:205–209

Dewhurst C J (ed) 1981 Integrated obstetrics and gynaecology for postgraduates, 3rd edn. Blackwell Scientific Publications, Oxford, p 536

Dmowski W P 1980 Symposium: finding the best therapy for endometriosis. Contemporary Obstetrics and Gynaecology 15:81

Ernst A, Aguilera E, Dabancens A 1981 Alteration of the physiology of the fallopian tubes by endosalpingiosis. Reproduction 5:87–93

Fathalla M F 1967 Malignant transformation in ovarian endometriosis. Journal of Obstetrics and Gynaecology of the British Commonwealth 74:85–92

Fianu S, Ingelman-Sunberg A, Nasiell K, Rosen J, Vaclauinkeva U 1980 Surgical treatment of post abortion endometriosis of the bladder and post-operative bladder function. Scandinavian Journal of Urology and Nephrology 14:151–155

Furman W R, Wang K P, Summer W R, Tery P D 1980 Catamenial pneumothorax evaluation by fibroptic pleuroscopy. American Review of Respiratory Disease 121:137–140

Gantt P A, Hunt J B, McDonough P G 1981 Progestin reversal of ureteral endometriosis. Obstetrics and Gynecology 57:665–667

Gardner B, Whittaker R H 1981 The use of danazol for ureteral obstruction caused by endometriosis. Journal of Urology 125:117–118

Gini P C, Chukudebelu W O, Onigbo W I B 1981 Perforation of the appendix during pregnancy, a rare complication of pregnancy. British Journal of Obstetrics and Gynaecology 88:456–458

Grimes D A, Fowler W C 1980 Adeno-squamous carcinoma of the caecum arising in endometriosis. Gynaecological Oncology 9:254–255

Guzick D S, Bross D S, Rock J A 1982 Assessing the efficiency of the American fertility society's classification of endometriosis, application of a dose response methodology. Fertility and Sterility 38:171–176

Endometriosis

Hassan H M 1981 Classifications for endometriosis. Fertility and Sterility 35:368–369

Hibbard L T, Schumann W R, Goldstein G E 1981 Thoracic endometriosis: a review and report of 2 cases. American Journal of Obstetrics and Gynecology 140:227–232

Honore L H 1980 Endometriosis of Meckel's diverticulum associated with intestinal obstruction. American Journal of Proctology 31:11–12

Joel-Cohen S J 1978 The place of the abdominal hysterectomy. Clinics in Obstetrics and Gynaecology 5:525–543

Jurewicz W A, Brough W A, Whittaker R A, Wheeler T R 1983 Atypical (endometrial) carcinoma of the prostate. Journal of the Royal Society of Medicine 76:372–373

Kistner R W, Siegel A M, Behrman S J 1977 Suggested classification for endometriosis and relationship to infertility. Fertility and Sterility 78:10008–1010

Langman J, Rowland R, Vernon-Roberts B 1981 Endometriosis of the appendix. British Journal of Surgery 2:121–124

Mackay E V, Beischer W, Cox L W, Wood C 1983 Illustrated textbook of gynaecology, W B Saunders and Co, Sydney, p 241

Malinak L R 1980 Infertility and endometriosis: operative techniques staging and prognosis. Clinical Obstetrics and Gynecology 23:925–936

Mettler L 1982 Pathology of endometriosis. In: Semm K, Greenblatt R, Mettler L (eds) Genital endometriosis in infertility. Georg Thieme Verlag, Stuttgart, p 11–20

Meyer W, Sailer R, Vandenhorst W, Lenz D, Breuer W 1980 Chirurgische therapie aer bickdarm—endometriosis. Munchener Medizinische Wochen Schrift 112:415–518

Moore J G, Hibbard L T, Growdon W A, Shifrin B S 1979 Urinary tract endometriosis: enigmas in diagnosis and management. American Journal of Obstetrics and Gynecology 134:162–172

Mostoufizadeh M, Scully R E 1980 Malignant tumours arising in endometriosis. Clinical Obstetrics and Gynecology 23:957–963

Pillay S P, Hardie I R 1980 Intestinal complications of endometriosis. British Journal of Surgery 67:677–679

Pittaway D E 1983 Appendicectomy in the surgical treatment of endometriosis. Obstetrics and Gynecology 61:421–424

Pittaway D E, Daniell J H, Maxson W S, Winfield A C, Wentz A C 1982 Recurrence of ureteral obstruction caused by endometriosis after danazol therapy. American Journal of Obstetrics and Gynecology 145:720–722

Pittaway D, Marson W, Daniell J, Herbert C, Wentz A C 1983 Luteal phase defects in infertility patients with endometriosis. Fertility and Sterility 39:712–713

Rock J A, Guzick D S, Sengos C, Schweditsch M, Sapik C, Jones H W Jr 1981 The conservative treatment of endometriosis, evaluation of pregnancy success with respect to extent of disease as categorized using contemporary classification system. Fertility and Sterility 35:131–137

Russell P 1979 The pathological assessment of ovarian neoplasms. I Introduction to the common epithelial tumours and analysis of benign epithelial tumours. Pathology 11:5–26

Sampson J A 1925 Endometrial carcinoma of the ovary arising in endometrial tissue in that organ. Archives of Surgery 10:15

Scully M S, Richardson G, Ballow J J 1966 The development of malignancy in endometriosis. Clinical Obstetrics and Gynaecology 9:384

Stenback F, Kaullila A 1981 Endometrioid ovarian tumours: morphology and relation to other endometrial conditions. Gynecologic and Obstetric Investigations 12:57–70

Stern H, Toole A L, Merino M 1980 Catamenial pneumothorax. Chest 78:480–482

Tulusan A H, Trotnow S 1983 Endometriotic ureteric obstruction after hysterectomy. Archives of Gynecology 232:149–151

Tutschka B G, Lauchlan S C 1980 Endosalpingiosis. Obstetrics and Gynecology 55:(suppl) 575–605

Williams T J, Pratt J H 1977 Endometriosis in 1000 conservative coeliotomies: incidence and management. American Journal of Obstetrics and Gynecology 129:245–250

Yamazaki S, Ogawa A J, Koide S, Shohzu A, Osamura Y 1980 Catamenial pneumothorax associated with endometriosis of the diaphragm. Chest 77:107–109

5

Clinical features and diagnosis

Traditionally it has been claimed that endometriosis can be diagnosed from a history of secondary or acquired dysmenorrhoea, dyspareunia, pelvic pain and infertility in a patient who, on vaginal examination, has a fixed, retroverted uterus, tender nodularity in the pouch of Douglas or around the utero-sacral ligaments, with or without ovarian enlargement or fixity.

Symptoms

The data from the Brisbane series were dissected by the computer and the information obtained on the occurrence of symptoms is shown in Table 5.1. A further sub-record analysis of these symptoms (Table 5.2) shows some interesting clustering of symptom complexes.

Table 5.1 Symptoms in order of occurrence in the Brisbane series

Dysmenorrhoea	227	Altered menstrual cycle	72
Dyspareunia	188	Pelvic mass	8
Nil	155	Bowel symptoms	3
Infertility	131	Bladder symptoms	2
Pelvic pain	114	Galactorrhoea	2
Menorrhagia	105		

No other symptom of significance occurred in more than one patient

Deductions made from these tables are that 155 of 717 patients (22%) had no symptoms while 39 of the 717 (5%) had all the significant symptoms of endometriosis—dysmenorrhoea, dyspareunia, pelvic pain and infertility.

Dysmenorrhoea

Most patients with dysmenorrhoea noticed a progressive alteration in the nature of their period pain, and altered timing of dysmenor-

Table 5.2 Symptom clusters in endometriosis

Symptom clusters	No. of patients
Dysmenorrhoea alone	66
Dyspareunia alone	48
Dysmenorrhoea + dyspareunia	48
Infertility alone	64
Pelvic pain alone	47
Pain + dysmenorrhoea	12
Pain + dyspareunia	18
Pain + dysmenorrhoea + dyspareunia	9
Pain + infertility	51
Infertility + dysmenorrhoea	83
Infertility + dyspareunia	61
Infertility + dysmenorrhoea + dyspareunia	37
Infertility + dysmenorrhoea + dyspareunia + pelvic pain	39

rhoea, which changed from premenstrual pain to pain commencing after the onset of bleeding and reaching a crescendo after a day or two of menstrual bleeding. This progressive change in the nature of dysmenorrhoea probably parallels the progressive damage caused by the disease. Endometriosis can produce dysmenorrhoea in the following ways:

1. Menstrual haemorrhage into an encysted space with increased intracystic pressure
2. Retrograde menstruation with peritoneal irritation
3. Increased prostaglandin production and release from ectopic secretory endometrium and from tissue damaged directly by endometriosis; this prostaglandin secretion causes local vasospasm and tissue anoxia, altered uterine and tubal motility, and increased magnitude of uterine contractions (Ben Nun & Greenblatt 1982)
4. Pain from neighbouring organs by direct irritation due to contact with endometrioma—for example bowel or bladder pain

Traditionally it was thought that dysmenorrhoea always altered with endometriosis but, in fact, the Brisbane series data show that 101 of the 227 females complaining of dysmenorrhoea had done so since the menarche. Many did not believe that the quality of pain had altered, only the quantity had worsened. A striking feature of the dysmenorrhoea present in the adolescent age group was that the majority (27 of 35) had had severe dysmenorrhoea since the menarche, and this was significant in the decisions made about the management of adolescents with dysmenorrhoea. A girl complaining of severe dysmenorrhoea since the menarche with no abatement would be most likely to undergo laparoscopic investigation.

It is certainly difficult to quantify the very subjective symptom of dysmenorrhoea. Individual pain tolerance, the location and severity of the disease, and cultural attitudes to menstruation, all play significant roles. In the Republic of Vanuatu where native medicine men used many counterirritants such as inflicting superficial burns with hot sticks and hot coals to ease pain, including dysmenorrhoea, it was common to find multiple superficial burn scars or keloids on the torso and thighs of women suffering from dysmenorrhoea, which was often due to either chronic pelvic inflammatory disease, endometriosis, or malignant disease. One of the difficulties in treating patients in that area for these diseases was 'local custom'. For instance, sexually transmitted diseases were regarded by 'local custom' as only of importance in the male members of the community and women consequently were seldom seen in the acute phase when appropriate orthodox antibiotic therapy would be of maximal value to them.

In her review of dysmenorrhoea, Sobczyk (1980) noted that one of the five psychological forces operating when women seek medical care, is anticipation of a return of good health. Many women do not believe dysmenorrhoea is a sign of bad health. Many believe it is an abnormality for which there is no cure. Many are disheartened by previously prescribed therapies that have proved ineffective and are therefore reluctant to seek further help, and regard their plight as hopeless.

One fact that became obvious during the years of the Brisbane series survey was that all women, irrespective of age, having dysmenorrhoea, irrespective of quality and quantity, that does not respond to simple analgesics or antiprostaglandins should be laparoscoped to exclude endometriosis, especially in the adolescent years, when dysmenorrhoea is sufficient to incapacitate them periodically with respect to school, work, or play. It is rare for idiopathic dysmenorrhoea to cause prolonged progressive incapacity in the absence of serious and obvious psychological problems. No woman should be labelled as psychologically disturbed, however, until laparoscopy at least has been employed to exclude endometriosis.

Patients experiencing menstrual tenesmus or strangury should also be fully investigated to exclude endometriosis with involvement of bowel and/or bladder. Endometriosis involving the left ovary commonly causes periodic disturbances of emptying of the sigmoid colon which may be the only symptom and if full gastroenterological investigation rules out intramural or intraluminal bowel disease, laparoscopy should be performed to exclude endometriosis.

Dyspareunia

Of the 717 patients in the Brisbane series, 668 were or had been sexually active and of the sexually active women, 188 (28%) admitted to dyspareunia. Like urinary incontinence, dyspareunia is a symptom to which many women are reluctant to admit because of imagined defectiveness in their femininity if such problems are acknowledged. Alternatively some women deny experiencing pain with intercourse but then conceded on further questioning that they attempt coitus only in certain positions having found previously that other postures or positions produced significant coital pain.

Any coital posture that facilitates deep penetration and associated stretching of the uterine supports may produce dysparaeunia in endometriosis and other pathological states. However, although 5 out of 7 women in the Brisbane series had endometriosis involving the pouch of Douglas and uterosacral ligament area, and although nearly 5 out of 7 had a major degree of endometriosis, it seems remarkable that only 1 in 4 of the sexually active females admitted to dysparenia even on close direct questioning.

No symptoms

A total of 155 (22%) patients had no symptoms. Most of these patients were diagnosed quite coincidentally during surgical procedures for other conditions e.g. laparoscopic sterilizations. However, about one-half had positive signs and again these were detected during examination for other symptom complexes—abnormal cytology, urinary incontinence etc.

Infertility

There is a marked concern in contemporary literature about infertility and endometriosis and, indeed, the interlocking mutually significant aetiological factors, the mutually dependent therapeutic outcomes etc. have all been noted. However, in the Brisbane series only 131 patients with a diagnosis of endometriosis specifically complained of infertility at the time of consultation. Of these, 101 had primary infertility, 24 had secondary infertility and six patients have been treated elsewhere for secondary infertility including two who were unsuccessfully treated by in vitro fertilization elsewhere, and four who were habitual aborters still complaining of failure of success. Of the 131 with the complaint of infertility, 64 had no other symptoms and of this 64 only 11 had no signs.

Thus, 11 of 131 infertile women in a total group of 717 patients had neither other symptoms nor signs, a very small percentage indeed.

During the course of this study other patients also developed infertility so later considerations of treatment effectiveness will show a larger number of infertile patients than the 131 who specifically complained of infertility at the time of the initial consultation. The incidence of endometriosis in infertile patients in this practice is 271 of 530 patients (51%)—a high incidence probably biased for the reasons mentioned previously.

Pelvic pain

Non-specific pelvic pain occurred in 114 of the 717 patients (16%) in the Brisbane series. This was pain that was not periodic, did not resemble dysmenorrhoea, yet interfered with the patients' lifestyles sufficiently to require regular analgesics, or even caused incapacity or inability to perform normal functions. Reviewing the laparoscopic findings in 1194 consecutive diagnostic laparoscopies performed for pelvic pain, Cunanen et al (1983) noted 511 (42.8%) had had previous pelvic surgery.

Preoperative pelvic examination in their series revealed no signs in 749 cases, and 479 of these (64%) were found to have abnormalities diagnosed at laparoscopy. On the other hand, 445 patients had abnormal findings on pelvic examination but at operation 78 (17.5%) had no abnormality detected.

Therefore, the diagnostic error when relying on clinical examination alone in symptomatic patients was from 17.5 to 64%.

The age range in their series was 15–80 years (mean 29 years) and the parity was 0–7 (mean 3+). They used the classic criteria for pelvic inflammatory disease, namely:

1. Tubal hyperaemia and congestion
2. Pus in the fimbrial end of the tube
3. Hydrosalpinges
4. Adnexal adhesions

In this regard the Brisbane series corresponded. These researchers also found 43 cases of endometriosis in their series, a very low incidence compared with the Brisbane series and they noted that 51% (22 out of 43) had abnormal pelvic findings while 49% (21 out of 43) were reported as clinically normal. In similar fashion, of eight ectopic pregnancies in their series, three were reported as clinically normal on pelvic examination. The point to be made here is that while it is acknowledged that ectopic pregnancy is difficult to diagnose accurately on clinical examination alone, the same holds true for endometriosis.

In the majority of the patients in the Brisbane series with pelvic pain, the pain was inflammatory in origin, and in a group of 47 who complained of pain only, most were referred by other specialists, for example gastroenterologists, for laparoscopy because diagnostic efforts to ascribe the pain to the bowel had proven negative. Of course, in some patients pain and a complaint of a mass were indeed due to the so-called 'irritable colon' syndrome, but not only may endometriosis coexist with this distressing disease, it may also initiate it if the endometriosis is on or near the bowel or its investing peritoneum.

Menorrhagia

Again this is a difficult symptom to quantify and qualify although Fraser et al (1983) claimed that a measured blood loss at menses in excess of 80 ml was diagnostic of menorrhagia. In the Brisbane series patients in whom menstrual loss was so heavy as to produce anaemia, cause interference with normal lifestyles, or incapacity and confinement indoors for fear of embarrassment during menstruation, were regarded as having menorrhagia.

Of the 15% of the Brisbane series patients experiencing this symptom, almost all had other coexistent disease entities such as adenomyosis, fibroids, pelvic inflammatory disease, or polycystic ovary disease. In these cases the menorrhagia is probably unrelated to endometriosis and it is likely it would have been a problem even if endometriosis had not been present. There were many instances where a hysterectomy was performed for menorrhagia and endometriosis was only coincidentally diagnosed at operation.

Altered menstrual cycle

One unusual patient in the Brisbane series had only one symptom, namely two years of secondary amenorrhoea. The amenorrhoea developed after she started competitive long-distance foot racing. Recent research suggests that such women have prostaglandin secretions at variance with the norm, but there is nothing to suggest that endometriosis in this woman was related to her new found physical activities. Although her uterus had involuted to approximately $2 \times 2 \times 1$ cm in size, there was no suggestion that her endometriosis had undergone similar involutions.

Patients with oligomenorrhoea were usually those who had concomitant polycystic ovary disease and there were an additional 26 patients presenting with oligomenorrhoea after cessation of combined oral contraceptive therapy. Those patients taking oral contraceptives at the time of diagnosis of endometriosis (113) would be expected to have little in the way of menstrual cycle disturbance so that the incidence would seem to be 72 patients out of a corrected total of 597 (12%) complaining of disturbed menstrual cycles. The number 597 is obtained by subtracting from the total of 717 the 113 on oral contraception, together with the six patients in the series who had previously undergone hysterectomy and the one patient whose ovaries had both been removed previously.

Galactorrhoea

A distinct 'Galactorrhoea-Endometriosis' syndrome has been proposed by Hirschowitz et al (1978). These workers had a remarkable group of nine women with endometriosis and galactorrhoea. They also had 30 other women with galactorrhoea and no endometriosis attending their clinic for endocrine studies. Seven of the patients with endometriosis plus galactorrhoea were nulliparous and five had galactorrhoea at the initial consultation. Several also had polycystic ovary syndrome. None had elevated prolactin levels and three of seven given danazol therapy of 400 mg daily developed galactorrhoea. A further three who had galactorrhoea prior to this therapy were not changed by it. In all cases when the endometriosis was controlled, galactorrhoea subsided. These authors were unable to explain this 'syndrome'.

The fact that only two patients of the 717 in the Brisbane series complained of galactorrhoea suggests that the syndrome is a fairly tenuous concept. In the Brisbane series a further two patients developed galactorrhoea while on Depo-provera therapy: both are pregnant at the time of writing and the galactorrhoea has ceased with cessation of progestogen therapy.

Corenblum and Taylor (1982) have also suggested that the reported link between endometriosis, polycystic ovary disease and hyperprolactinaemia–galactorrhoae needs further clarification. Certainly normo-prolactinaemic galactorrhoea is far more common in Brisbane.

Premenstrual spotting

Premenstrual spotting was not specifically investigated in the Brisbane series. However, Anne Colston Wentz (1980) reported that eight of 23 patients (35%) diagnosed as having endometriosis complained of premenstrual spotting for three or more days each month. She did not find this phenomenon to be related to luteal phase deficiency as previously reported, and it was not, in her experience, related to progesterone deficiency. The exact relationship remains obscure.

Signs

The data obtained in Tables 5.1 and 5.3 when cross checked on the computer produced the interesting information that only 33 of the 717 patients in the Brisbane series had neither symptoms nor signs—that is 5%.

Table 5.3 Signs found in order of occurrence in the Brisbane series

Uterine tenderness	220	
Uterine enlargement	213	
Pouch of Douglas nodules	205	
Ovarian tenderness	152	(unilateral 130)
Ovarian enlargement	146	(unilateral 123)
Uterine retroversion—fixed	121	
Retroverted uterus—mobile	103	
Nil	96	
Pelvic mass	19	
'Acute abdomen'	18	
Recto-vaginal septum nodules	13	
Congenital anomaly	4	
Vaginal disease	4	
Cervical stenosis	2	

No signs

While one would anticipate a significant number of stage 0 and stage I patients who would not show any signs, in fact a computer review of the Brisbane series showed two stage IV patients who had had surgery for other reasons and in whom a frozen pelvis due to endometriosis was discovered at operation, both these patients having been recorded as having no gynaecological signs. There were a further five patients with considerable destructive changes which were not recognized on clinical examination, although the author is obsessively interested in finding endometriosis. It is unusual to find no signs suggestive of endometriosis even when there are no symptoms, and obesity is the major common contributing factor to negative findings in those mentioned cases, especially in those who have coincidental polycystic ovary disease and endometriosis.

Uterine signs

Uterine tenderness in 220 (31%) and uterine enlargement in 213 (29%), are curious findings in a disease process where diagnostic location of the disease (Table 4.1) showed that the uterus was involved in only 67 of 717 patients with endometriosis. As mentioned in relation to menorrhagia, it is possible that coincidental findings of fibroids and adenomyosis would favour uterine enlargement and tenderness. Despite this there were many patients in whom these signs of tenderness and enlargement were unexplained.

Nodularity and tenderness in pouch of Douglas and rectovaginal septum

These signs were found in 228 (31%) of patients in the Brisbane series, and vaginal, rectal or combined rectovaginal examination as recommended by Kistner (1975) can be used with effect in the sexually active patient to clarify these signs. Gentleness is required, however, as this approach usually also confirms the location of dyspareunia trigger areas and painful nodules and one hopes to avoid hurting the patient and possibly driving her away from further care because of an unpleasant confrontation experience. Examination at the time of menstruation was recommended by Kistner for accurate determination and location of endometriomata and certainly laparoscopy examination at this time can be most rewarding.

It is often difficult to determine whether lesions are nodules in the true rectovaginal septum or whether they represent isolated endometriomata located in scar tissue consequent on the gradual occlusion and obliteration of the pouch of Douglas. It matters little in terms of symptoms and management although lesions in this location provide a useful guide to response to non-surgical treatment.

Uterine retroversion

In 121 patients in the Brisbane series (17%) a fixed uterine retroversion was a positive finding. In a further 103 patients (14%) a mobile retroversion was found and the significance of this is obscure since the oft stated incidence of one in five women showing uterine retroversion in the absence of disease, has never been validated in Brisbane. While TeLinde & Scott (1951) found uterine retroversion favoured the development of endometriosis due to retrograde menstrual spill, there are many women in the community with a mobile retroversion and no endometriosis.

Fixed retroversion is believed to result from endometriotic scar tissue contraction following obliteration of the pouch of Douglas by endometriosis and, in the same way, many other patients develop a fixed anteversion with scarring from endometriosis in the utero-vesical fold and round ligaments. It is the 'fixity' rather than the uterine position that is the diagnostic clue and fixity suggests that the disease has progressed beyond stage I, and this is important in planning and individualizing the diagnostic, surgical and therapeutic attack.

The 'acute abdomen'

In only 18 cases were the presenting signs due to acute peritoneal irritation and in five of these an ectopic pregnancy was the direct cause. In the other 13 cases a mixture of conditions ranging from acute appendicitis in a non-endometriomatous appendix to endometriotic adhesive small gut obstruction were present.

In only one case was the acute problem due to a ruptured endometrial cyst—this followed a vigorous vaginal examination by an enthusiastic colleague at the time of taking a routine Papanicolasu smear in a patient who was asymptomatic. There was no case of spontaneous rupture of an endometriotic cyst.

In most of the 'acute abdomen' cases infection was the commonest finding and often laparoscopic examination had been performed to exclude an ectopic pregnancy. In many cases of pelvic inflammation, a routine leucocyte count and ESR proved to be of little value, being reported as normal on many occasions when laparoscopy showed acute salpingitis or even purulent peritonitis, sometimes coexistent with endometriosis.

Adnexal signs

It is obvious therefore that laparoscopic examination was necessary to determine the cause of adnexal tenderness (21% of cases) and enlargement (20%) in patients with endometriosis because the most dangerous possibilities that might have required urgent intervention were neoplastic changes on the one hand, and ectopic pregnancy on the other.

Diagnosis

All 717 patients in the Brisbane series had surgery involving inspection of endometriosis and staging of disease process. The diagnostic operations performed in the first instance are shown in Table 5.4. The patients diagnosed at vaginal repair operation posed

Table 5.4 Diagnostic operations in the Brisbane series

Laparoscopy	414
Laparotomy	111
Hysterectomy	168
Caesarean section	12
Vaginal repair	8
Hernia repair	2
Cervical biopsy	1
Excisions vaginal tumour	1
Total	717

a special problem. When the utero-vesical fold and/or pouch of Douglas peritoneum were opened and unsuspected endometriosis discovered, the problem became one of whether it is justifiable to rely on what can be visualized of the adnexa, pelvic peritoneum, bladder surface and visible bowel surface through the peritoneal incision, or whether a coincidental laparotomy is necessary or justified. Obviously individual judgement is required and if the disease if stage I or even localized stage II then it may be justifiable to not proceed immediately to laparotomy, but to use postoperative medication to arrest the disease process after fulguration of visible lesions through the open vaginal vault.

Obviously destruction of the normal peritoneum and pouch of Douglas anatomy is an absolute contraindication to continuing with vaginal surgery and an abdominal approach either then or later, is mandatory.

Oak et al (1983) stated clearly that definitive diagnosis of endometriosis is only possible by direct visualization at laparoscopy or laparotomy with which the author totally agrees. At that diagnostic procedure staging or classification should also be carried out using some simple diagram of the internal pelvic organs (Fig. 5.1) and related bowel and bladder. On such a diagram operative findings, staging, and location of disease are recorded.

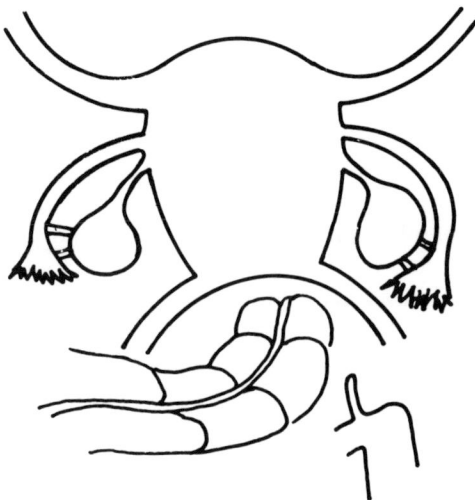

Fig. 5.1 Diagram used to record operative findings for endometriosis

Peritoneal flushing and cytology

The need to find a suitable screening system for detecting early endometriosis led Portuondo et al (1982) to evaluate exfoliative cytology by sampling peritoneal washings and matching results with subsequent laparoscopic endometriosis biopsy. The correlation was poor as in only 25% of cases of endoscopically proven endometriosis were the peritoneal washings cytologically diagnostic for endometriosis.

Ultrasound examination

Sandler & Karo (1978) mentioned the shaggy irregular ultrasonic appearance of the wall of endometriotic cysts and the difficulty in distinguishing between pelvic inflammatory disease, simple ovarian cysts, and ovarian malignancy by ultrasound examination. Goldman & Minkin (1980) admitted that there is no specific ultrasound pattern for endometriosis. There seems to be at present a trend in primary care practitioners to order gynaecological ultrasound screening examination in women with gynaecological symptoms sometimes before they have even done a physical examination. Not only is the diagnostic yield in the non-pregnant patient relatively poor, but the expense involved is high and the possibility of a mischievous false positive finding occurring cannot be ruled out. The author knows one patient who presented with dysmenorrhoea in her late teens and before pelvic examination was carried out she had an ultrasound examination of her pelvis performed by a radiologist. He reported abnormal findings on the left side of the pelvis and suggested a pelvic computerized axial tomography scan. This was performed almost immediately and led him to sign a report stating that this young girl had a significant area of her lower uterine cavity occupied by cancer. When subsequent physical examination and diagnostic curettage excluded any abnormality whatsoever, the emotional anguish inflicted on this girl and her family were in no way relieved but, in fact, led to them doubting the accuracy of the ultimate histological report! This is a significant true example of the extent to which esoteric investigations may intrude into the world of common sense in medical practice.

Nuclear magnetic resonance imaging

Nuclear magnetic resonance (NMR) utilizes radio frequency radiation. Varying magnetic fields are used to produce cross-sectional images of the body including the pelvic organs. The image depends on the number of hydrogen nuclei in the tissues scanned and the extent to which these nuclei are bound within each organic molecule. This technique is non-invasive and avoids the use of potentially dangerous ionizing radiation so is without apparent hazard. The image plane is electronically selected and direct coronal, sagittal, and transverse images can be used.

Johnson et al (1984) reported enthusiastically the results of a small trial which included a patient with bilateral ovarian endometriosis. The NMR images from this patient were of high density which reflected the blood and lipid-rich material contents of the endometrial cysts. The authors suggest this distinctive appearance could lead to NMR becoming a useful non-invasive diagnostic tool in endometriosis because they believe small deposits could also be picked up because of the high density of such endometriotic lesions.

Future developments are awaited with a healthy scepticism. Since one swallow does not make a summer, one case of bilateral endometriosis of the ovary scanned by NMR does not make a new ideal diagnostic procedure for endometriosis.

Laparoscopy

There is no justification for entering the peritoneal cavity in a diagnostic capacity in the management of endometriosis unless lesions can be fully visualized, biopsied, and staged.

A most significant milestone in the author's life pilgrimage was when Professor Eric Mackay of the University of Queensland, introduced him to the laparoscope in Brisbane in February 1967. In the following month we performed the first diagnostic laparoscopy in this part of the world and a year later had the singularly exciting privilege of sharing a week's work with Patrick Steptoe, who generously shared his knowledge and experience with us in Brisbane, thus paving the way for surgical procedures to be done laparoscopically. Many colleagues were slow to accept the legitimacy of laparoscopy for a long time, but now this procedure is so universally routine that there is no need to discuss further matters of the history of the procedure or questions of technique or complications, save to say that in the Brisbane series in the early days especially, the enthusiastic cooperation and wise advice of Dr Walter Biggs, specialist anaesthetist who has anaesthetized most of the patients in the Brisbane series, has played a major role in the successes achieved. It was Dr Biggs who in 1968 suggested the simple inexpensive but safe pneumoperitoneum technique still used and his preparedness to alter the position of the anaesthetized patient both on the operating table and in space has facilitated biopsy and surgical techniques at laparoscopy.

The confidential report into gynaecological laparoscopy released by the Royal College of Obstetricians and Gynaecologists (RCOG) in London in 1978 has established the safety of laparoscopy and in a survey of 50 000 laparoscopies they noted a complication rate of 3.6% irrespective of all factors including the status of the surgeon or anaesthetist.

In the author's practice of 6656 patients 1639 laparoscopies were performed and endometriosis was diagnosed in 414—an incidence of 25% which is comparable to that of Riedel & Semm (1982) who found endometriosis in 26% of 6200 laparoscopic examinations. Prior to the reintroduction of laparoscopy in the USA in the 1960s Cohen (1980) noted that stage I–II endometriosis was seldom diagnosed, while Corson (1979) suggested that Eward's report of 1978 and his results in treating infertility patients with stage I–II endometriosis influenced gynaecologists from the USA to emulate European and Australian colleagues in performing surgical procedures at laparoscopy.

Laparoscopy is an invasive diagnostic procedure and therefore potentially hazardous. Certain constant factors have been observed in the Brisbane series:

1. Diagnostic laparoscopy is performed as an inpatient procedure using aseptic techniques without abdominal shaving
2. General anaesthesia expertly administered, usually with endotracheal intubation and positive pressure ventilation is utilized
3. Biopsies and fulguration, where applicable, are carried out through a second portal of entry using Semm's ancillary equipment (Semm & Mettler 1980)
4. At the same time coincidental surgical procedures as required are performed: ventrosuspension (Patterson et al 1978); aspiration of ovarian cysts; needle biopsy of ovaries; uterine curettage; hydrotubation for tubal patency assessment
5. The relatively avascular incisions which, because of a constant awareness for the need to inflict minimal scarring on these patients, are placed in the lower umbilicus for laparoscopy, and in the midline of the upper margin of the pubic hair line for the second portal of entry
6. All the surfaces of all the pelvic organs must be displayed for diagnostic accuracy and this applies especially to the ovary which must be lifted with grasping forceps so that its undersurface can be inspected if laparoscopy is to be truly diagnostic.

Diagnosis at laparotomy, hysterectomy, and other operations

It would be dishonest to suggest that endometriosis had been foremost in the surgeon's mind at the time of these other 303 diagnostic operations in the Brisbane series. Obviously this was not so, although where such problems as menorrhagia with obvious fibroids and a fixed tender pelvic tumour with severe dysmenorrhoea and dyspareunia were the indications for open operation, endometriosis was a definite consideration.

The laparotomy group included a subset of 13 patients having myomectomy operations for infertility, recurrent abortion and so on, who were found to have coincidental endometriosis, and several of the hysterectomy patients also became hysterectomies during the course of a laparotomy when it was found that a combination of endometriosis and another disease such as fibroids caused such surgical problems as to be 'non-salvageable'. The group of 12 patients in whom endometriosis was diagnosed at Caesarean section are another interesting subgroup because in only three of them was endometriosis suspected prior to conception. In all cases the disease was at least stage II and in three it was shown to have progressed on review at second-look surgery despite lactational amenorrhoea from 4 to 9 months in all cases. In keeping with the policy of dealing with endometriosis when discovered because it is often domestically, financially, and geographically difficult for patients to return for example, up to 1000 miles or so to Brisbane for further surgery, all these patients had conservative surgery performed at the time of Caesarean section. Seven of them have subsequently had successful pregnancies with no sign of recurrence and three have been lost to follow up.

Differential diagnosis

The only safe, reliable way to distinguish between endometriosis, pelvic inflammatory disease, pelvic neoplasm, and disorders of gastrointestinal, urological, and neurological systems that may produce similar symptoms or signs to endometriosis, is by laparoscopy or laparotomy.

No infertile female should be denied laparoscopy, and a careful search for endometriosis when no other cause for infertility or pelvic pain can be found, is mandatory. Other diagnostic procedures are ineffective—ultrasound is non-invasive but unreliable, radiography has no value greater than that of direct vision at surgery, peritoneal lavage and cytology examination is totally unreliable, and on the basis of one documented case, nuclear magnetic resonance may hold some magic potential for the future as a non-invasive diagnostic technique.

Endometriosis

REFERENCES

Ben Nun I, Greenblatt R B 1982 In: Semm K, Greenblatt R B, Mettler L (eds) Genital endometriosis in infertility. Thiem Stratton Inc, New York, p 3

Cohen M R 1980 Laparoscopic diagnosis and pseudomenopause treatment of endometriosis with danazol. Clinical Obstetrics and Gynaecology 23:902–915

Corenblum B, Taylor 1982 The hyperprolactinaemic polycystic ovary syndrome may not be a distinct entity. Fertility and Sterility 38:549–552

Corson S 1979 Use of the laparoscope in the infertile patient. Fertility and Sterility 32:359–369

Cunanen R G, Courey N G, Lippes J 1983 Laparoscopic findings in patients with pelvic pain. American Journal of Obstetrics and Gynecology 146:589–591

Eward D R 1978 Cauterization of stage I and II endometriosis and the resulting pregnancy rate. In: Phillips J (ed) Endoscopy in gynecology. American Association of Gynaeocological Laparoscopists, California, USA, p 276–278

Fraser I S, McCarron G, Markham K, Robinson M, Smythe E 1983 Long term treatment of menorrhagia with mefenamic acid. Obstetrics and Gynecology 61:109–112

Goldman S M, Minkin S I 1980 Diagnosing endometriosis with ultrasound. Accuracy and specificity. Journal of Reproductive Medicine 25:178–182

Hirshowitz J S, Soler R G, Worstman J 1978 The galactorrhoea–endometriosis syndrome. Lancet 1:896–898

Johnson I R, Symonds E M, Worthington B S et al 1984 Imaging ovarian tumours by nuclear magnetic resonance. British Journal of Obstetrics and Gynaecology 91:260–264

Kistner R W 1975 Management of endometriosis in the infertile patient. Fertility and Sterility 26:1151–1161

Oak M K, Williams C A U, Elstein M 1983 The current status of infertility associated with pelvic endometriosis. Clinical Reproduction and Fertility 2:97–112

Paterson M E L, Jordan J A, Logan-Edwards R 1978 A survey of 100 patients who had laparoscopic ventrosuspensions. British Journal of Obstetrics and Gynaecology 85:468

Portuondo J A, Herran C, Echanojaurgei A D, Riego A G 1982 Peritoneal flushing and biopsy in laparoscopically diagnosed endometriosis. Fertility and Sterility 38:538–541

Riedel H H, Semm K 1982 Mechanism and influence of antigonadotrophin treatment with danazol: clinical experiences with a 3-step therapy for extragenital endometriosis. In: Semm K, Greenblatt R B, Mettler L (eds) Genital endometriosis in infertility. Thieme Stratton, New York, p. 43

RCOG 1978 Gynaecological laparoscopy: the report of the Working Party of the Confidential Enquiry into Gynaecological Laparoscopy. Chamberlain G, Carron Brown J (eds) Royal College of Obstetricians and Gynaecologists, London

Sandler M A, Karo J J 1978 The spectrum of ultrasound findings in endometriosis. Radiology 127:229–231

Semm K, Mettler L 1980 Technical progress in pelvic surgery via operative laparoscopy. American Journal of Obstetrics and Gynecology 138:121–127

Sobczyk R 1980 Dysmenorrhoea, the neglected syndrome. Journal of Reproductive Medicine 25:198–200

TeLinde R W, Scott R B 1951 External endometriosis. Clinical and experimental. American Surgeon 17:394–405

Wentz A C 1980 Premenstrual spotting: its association with endometriosis with no luteal phase inadequacy. Fertility and Sterility 33:605–607

6

Treatment of endometriosis

In the management of endometriosis mandatory individualization of treatment programmes depends on the patient's age, the extent and severity of the endometriosis, previous pelvic surgery, fertility requirements (immediate, completed, or to be deferred), and the patient's overall wishes.

After considering the given facts concerning the severity and extent of their endometriosis, some women may opt for no active treatment in the face of severe disease, or may prefer radical treatment for relatively minor disease, and such a choice is legitimate, provided it is based on complete factual knowledge and understanding of the problem.

While infertility is an emotive aspect of endometriosis, it is not a problem or a priority for all patients. Because pregnancy offers an easily measured response to therapy, most published works concentrate on pregnancy outcome as a cure indicator whatever the treatment programme (Buttram 1979a, Sadigh et al 1977, Rock et al 1981). Rantala et al (1983) reported a mean pregnancy rate after surgery in 129 infertile patients with endometriosis of 51.2%—after primary infertility 48.9%, after secondary infertility 56.8%. They found that two-thirds of these patients conceived within one year after surgery and the best results of surgery occurred when it was performed on patients with infertility of less than 5 years' duration. Using the Acosta staging system, the results were pregnancy rates of 59.1% in mild, 56.4% in moderate, and 40% in severe endometriosis.

Other workers have published recent studies questioning the value of active interference in endometriosis in terms of pregnancy outcome. Garcia & David (1977), reported 17 cases of mild endometriosis where conception occurred without any active treatment within 2 years of diagnosis. Portuondo et al (1983) quoted a 61.2% accumulative pregnancy rate within 18 months of surgical diagnosis of endometriosis without active interference. Schenken & Malinak (1982), comparing expectant management with conservative surgery in patients with mild endometriosis, found pregnancy rates of 75% and 74.2% respectively in these groups, suggesting that it is justifiable to defer active intervention in mild endometriosis where pregnancy is desired immediately. This issue has been further thrown open by the analysis of pregnancy outcome in 1145 infertile couples (Collins et al 1983). These workers analysed a 2–7 year follow-up of this large group of infertile couples to determine the frequency of pregnancy occurring independently of any treatment administered. Pregnancy occurred in 246 of 597 treated couples (41%) and in 191 of 548 untreated couples (35%). However, in the treated group 31% of pregnancies occurred more than 3 months after the last medical treatment, or more than 12 months after adnexal surgical treatment. These pregnancies, together with the 191 pregnancies in untreated couples, comprised 61% of all pregnancies and were defined as 'treatment-independent pregnancies'. In couples where there was an anovulatory defect, 44% fell into this category of 'treatment-independent' pregnancies as did 61% of pregnancies in couples with endometriosis, tubal defects or semen factors, and 96% of those couples with cervical factors or ideopathic infertility.

The conclusion drawn was that the potential for spontaneous cure in infertility is high. These workers suggested that there was a need for more ethically acceptable, randomized clinical trials of infertility treatment. It seems to be a justifiable argument that any active intervention programme in endometriosis management, irrespective of its effect on symptoms and signs, should be capable of producing a pregnancy rate in excess of 60% to compare with these results of expectant treatment, and to therefore be a justifiable management option. If it could be shown that 'treatment-independent pregnancy' effected a permanent cure of endometriosis, the argument for therapeutic inactivity might be sustainable. But we have no knowledge of the true incidence of endometriosis in the community, the spontaneous cure rate—if any, or the permanent cure rate after successful pregnancy—if at all.

The important 1983 publication of Wheeler & Malinak looked at recurrence of endometriosis. They found annual recurrence rates varying from 0.9% in the first year, up to 13.6% 8 years after treatment and the cumulative 3- and 5-year recurrence rates were 13.5% and 40.3% respectively. They found that pregnancy, while not preventing a recurrence, probably delayed the onset of recurrence.

Repeat conservative surgery was followed by pregnancy in 47% of their infertile patients and following a third conservative operation 20% of 20 infertile patients became pregnant. In this work the authors found no significant increase in the spontaneous abortion rate after treatment, in keeping with the Brisbane series, but curiously, in another study, Wheeler et al (1983) reported a fall in the spontaneous abortion rate from 34% to 9% following conservative therapy for endometriosis.

Obviously much more research into the significance of immune factors and immunocompetence together with the role of prostaglandins and their luteolytic function in the occurrence of spontaneous abortion in endometriosis needs to be carried out before the results of conservative surgical therapy in this situation can be truly assessed.

Depending on the extent of disease discovered at diagnostic operation, the management options utilized in the Brisbane series are outlined in Figure 6.1.

Surgical treatment

Conservative surgery

Laparoscopy

Laparoscopy has been a major surgical advance, not just in gynaecological diagnosis by ruling out the 'guess work factor', but in the operative surgical attack in less extensive cases of endometriosis, as well as other conditions predisposing to infertility or pelvic pain.

Following an instructive visit by Patrick Steptoe to Brisbane for a week in 1968, laparoscopy, which until then had only been diagnostic, became 'operative'. Initially unipolar electrocautery equipment was used but as soon as bipolar equipment became available it was utilized to increase the electrical safety factor and reduce the risk of undesirable adventitious electrical burns to neighbouring organs by directing the 240 V current through the electrical equipment and not through the patient, as with unipolar equipment.

Cohen (1982) writing of the almost epidemic incidence of endometriosis in American females from the menarche to the menopause, especially in those who were infertile, described how laparoscopy with visualization of the internal genitalia and the ability to perform biopsy, has enabled gynaecologists to make a definitive diagnosis much earlier in the disease process than

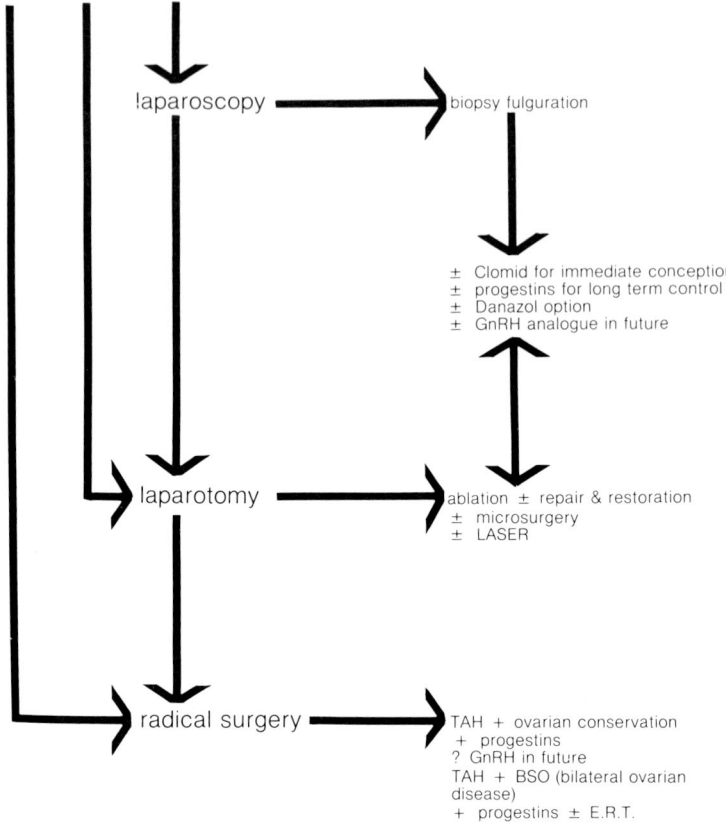

Fig. 6.1 Flow chart of management options utilized in the Brisbane series. TAH: total abdominal hysterectomy; BSO: bilateral salpingo-oopherectomy; GnRH: gonadotrophin releasing hormone; ERT: oestrogen replacement therapy

previously. He also suggested that treatment, medical, surgical or a combination of both, should commence at the time of diagnostic laparoscopy, a philosophy pursued since 1968 in the Brisbane series, especially in the younger patients with less extensive disease, who in most cases, have yet to put their fertility potential to the test.

The laparoscopic technique used in the Brisbane series varied little from that described by Steptoe in 1967 and the techniques of Frangenheim (1972) and Semm (1975) when performing electrocoagulation, were also only slightly modified. Patients are not routinely shaved, have no special bowel preparation, are anaesthetized and endotracheal intubation is used with positive pressure respiration. The bladder is emptied in the operating theatre following abdominal and vaginal preparation, midline incisions are used, at the inferior umbilical margin and at the upper pubic hair line, since the author prefers a two puncture technique for stereotactic ease of operating and safety. Others prefer a single entry technique. Indeed Sulewski et al (1980) reported 100 single puncture laparoscopic operations with unipolar fulguration and no mishaps. On the other hand, Millar (1978) suggested that while such laparoscopic diathermy procedures are tempting in the management of endometriosis deposits, the risks of damage to bowel or bladder made such surgery quite hazardous. The Brisbane series would suggest this is totally wrong if due care and skill are used, since no patient having laparoscopic surgery suffered any significant complication either intraperitoneal, thromboembolic, wound, or cardiorespiratory. Some patients did experience transient minor upper torso muscle ache from anaesthetic relaxing agent reaction or from residual intraperitoneal CO_2 irritating the undersurface of the diaphragm.

Diagnostic dilatation of the cervix to 6–7 mm combined with uterine curettage (D&C) was performed routinely in all cases at the time of laparoscopy. While Grimes & Peterson (1982) argued that the value of routine D&C has never been established, they believed that adding D&C to laparoscopy probably increased the morbidity of the operation at least twofold and that this increased morbidity plus the added expense and risks to the consumer outweighed any purported benefits. The most common complication noted in the Brisbane series was perforation of the uterine fundus with uterine sound (two cases), Hegar dilator (two cases) and small sharp curette (one case). None of these five perforations required treatment other than direct diathermy to control bleeding, three of them have been inspected at subsequent operations and no visible scar has been found, the other two patients have, between them, had five pregnancies and no further problems. Thus it seems that accidental uterine perforation at D&C may be a hazard, but in the absence of subsequent damage to other organs such as bowel, bladder or omentum, or the presence of gross infection (which would be a contraindication to such surgery anyhow) no long-term untoward sequelae seem likely.

Corson (1979) and Semm & Mettler (1980) have illustrated a comprehensive range of ancillary instruments for use at operative laparoscopy of which the most essential are holding and elevating forceps, electrocoagulation forceps and probe, biopsy forceps and scissors, and needle aspirators.

Additional surgical procedures can also be performed at laparoscopic operation for endometriosis; for example ovarian biopsy or needle aspiration of ovarian cysts, and ventrosuspension of the uterus when a retroversion is considered to be significant.

Portuondo et al (1982) preferred to carry out laparoscopic ovarian biopsy in their 230 infertile patients at about day 23 of the menstrual cycle in order to obtain more useful luteal phase information. They pointed out that, while this ovarian biopsy procedure might serve as a useful ovulation-inducing technique in polycystic ovary disease, it must be bloodless if peritubal or periovarian adhesions consequent on such surgery were to be avoided. Sutton (1974) had previously drawn attention to the risks in general, of post-ovarian biopsy haemorrhage in his series of 75 cases in which he used the Palmer drill forceps and electrocoagulation, as has been used in the Brisbane series.

Other significant sites of haemorrhage that can occur at laparoscopy and lead to fertility-compromising adhesions are the abdominal stab wounds. By keeping to the relatively avascular midline approach the author has found this to be no major problem in the Brisbane series, but occasionally it is necessary to use through and through nylon sutures to secure haemostatis of a stab wound, under laparoscopic vision, at either upper or lower wounds when inadvertent bleeding becomes a problem.

Ventrosuspension of a retroverted uterus can also be carried out at laparoscopy and the technique described by Paterson et al (1978) very closely followed that used in the Brisbane series since 1970. It requires nicety of judgement as to when to correct a uterine retroversion and, in general, asymptomatic retroversion in the absence of disease with obliteration of the pouch of Douglas, should be left alone. Ventrosuspension techniques in infertile patients utilizing plication of the round ligaments only, are to be avoided because they are more prone to produce intraperitoneal adhesions than techniques whereby the round ligament is drawn extraperitoneally and shortened by plication and attachment to the undersurface of the anterior rectus sheath.

Needle aspiration of simple cysts and the collection of cyst fluid for cytological examination to exclude neoplasm, and confirm the functional nature of most cysts, was also an additional part of laparoscopic surgery in the Brisbane series. Any patients with coexistent polycystic ovary disease were so treated by ovarian cyst drainage and diathermy. The services of a skilled cytologist helped to classify the various histological types encountered according to the presence or absence of granulosa cells, theca cells, or other cell types. A fringe benefit of such needle aspiration is that the occasional unsuspected intraovarian endometrioma will be revealed by needle aspiration of chocolate fluid and open operation can be carried out immediately. As mentioned previously in relation to polycystic ovary disease (PCOD) Gjönnaess (1984) has described a laparoscopic technique for ovarian electrocautery, a useful alternative to wedge resection of the ovary when PCOD and endometriosis coexist.

The importance of laparoscopic examination of all infertile patients, with or without symptoms of endometriosis, has been emphasized by Nordenskjold & Ahlgren (1983) and Moghissi & Wallach (1983). At least 50% of patients with negative clinical findings or normal hysterosalpingography, will have laparoscopically proven disease. Cunanan et al (1983) in an analysis of 3831 diagnostic laparoscopies, found 33% were performed for pelvic pain and 42% of the patients had had prior pelvic surgery. Of the 749 who were clinically 'normal', 63% had abnormal laparoscopic findings including 43 patients with endometriosis.

In 1978, Eward published the results of successful laparoscopic surgery in stage I and stage II endometriosis and since that time many others have been emboldened to emulate his work.

Now that laparoscopy is acknowledged as a legitimate gynaecological procedure and is more extensively available, it is not acceptable to diagnose endometriosis on purely clinical grounds. This fact has been recognized by the Australian Commonwealth Government which only subsidizes expensive drug therapy (danazol, dydrogesterone) when endometriosis has been surgically diagnosed (Jenkin 1980).

In the Brisbane series cost factors for these private patients have been constantly considered and no attempt has been made routinely to re-hospitalize patients for review laparoscopy following original surgery and/or medical therapy unless certain indications occurred such as:

1. Continued infertility 6 months or more after cessation of therapy where male factors are normal
2. Clinical progression of disease despite therapy
3. Before recommencing medical therapy where a previous 'cure' has re-presented with recurring symptoms or signs of endometriosis

Surrey & Breedman (1982) pointed out that the benefits to be derived from a second-look laparoscopy, particularly in patients who had had difficult pelvic surgery, included increased prognostic accuracy in assessing possible requirement for future therapy with recurrent endometriosis, the opportunity to learn by evaluation of individual surgical techniques, and the opportunity to perform fertility-enhancing procedures such as adhesiolysis, fimbrial dilatation, and cauterization of residual endometriomata. In their experience adhesions were the most common surgical complication in their 37 patients, and when the second-look laparoscopy was performed 6–8 weeks postoperatively the pregnancy rate was improved to 52%.

Since the formation of a successful fertility group in Brisbane, offering an in vitro fertilization (IVF) and embryo transfer (ET) service, laparoscopic assessment in the last 18 months has included the estimation of suitability of the patient, or more particularly the location and accessibility of the patient's ovaries, for possible future ovum collection, and IVF and ET.

The most important consideration confronting all operative laparoscopists is to know when not to attempt laparoscopic surgery. It is no disgrace to desist and proceed to laparotomy, either immediately or as a deferred procedure.

For the future, laparoscopy combined with laser therapy offers an exciting prospect in the treatment of endometriosis. Feste (1984) reported favourably on 44 of 158 patients with endometriosis treated with laparoscopy and laser in the USA while Sutton (1984) has used laser laparoscopy in a series of 60 patients in England.

Laparotomy

The decision to perform laparotomy, especially as a diagnostic procedure, was not necessarily related to endometriosis in the Brisbane series and the operative finding of endometriosis was sometimes merely a coincidental, unrelated finding to the disease causing presenting symptoms or signs.

In some cases, laparotomy led to immediate pelvic clearance, or hysterectomy with or without adnexal surgery, depending on the severity or stage of disease processes.

In two publications in 1979 (a & b) Buttram evaluated the place of conservative surgery in treating endometriosis—the treatment of choice for infertile women with endometriosis according to Andrews (1980). In the second paper Buttram described in detail surgical techniques used by him to achieve pregnancy rates of 73.2% in 88 mild, 55.9% in 50 moderate, and 40% in 68 severe cases of endometriosis. These stages of mild, moderate, and severe correlate with stages 1, 2 and 3 + 4 in the Brisbane series. Buttram emphasized that factors relating to his excellent success figures were:

1. When adnexal disease was unilateral he preferred excision of the involved unilateral organs rather than repair
2. Where conception was the immediate goal he advocated reduction in the likelihood of postoperative adhesions by judicious 'debulking', leaving diseased areas undisturbed when attempted excision or cauterization might predispose to tubo-ovarian adhesions. This is in keeping with the experience of Sadigh et al (1977) who had a 43% pregnancy rate in a group of infertile patients where attempts at resection of endometriosis in toto would have led to rectal resection and was therefore not pursued
3. The use of new suture materials of reduced biological reactivity (e.g. polyglycolic acid and polypropylene amide)
4. Reperitonealization after excision of endometriosis deposits with subsequent raw areas which could favour subsequent ooze of blood or serum and facilitate adhesion formation
5. Appendicectomy at the time of conservative surgery was deferred unless the appendix appeared to be the site of endometriosis.

Buttram also made use of presacral neurectomy, ventrosuspension, and plication of the utero-sacral ligaments in his approach to conservative surgical management.

Microsurgical principles are now universally accepted in conservative gynaecological surgical practice and infertility surgery (Gomel 1980). Gentle tissue handling, meticulous haemostasis, the use of superfine non-reactive suture materials, the use of an operating microscope and appropriate microsurgical instruments in operations planned in detail and performed in an unhurried atmosphere, will lead to superior surgical results, and probably the most significant trend in postgraduate surgical training will be to train more people in microsurgical principles and techniques.

One area where microsurgery may offer improved results is in those patients with tubal ectopic pregnancies. Pusey et al (1984) found that even with medical intervention obstetric performance after ectopic surgery was poor. These Canadian workers noted that Bronson (1977) claimed 50% of patients with an ectopic pregnancy had a subsequent successful outcome and Sherman et al (1982) noted that when there was a history of infertility followed by an ectopic pregnancy, then 53% of patients were subsequently successfully delivered. However, the Canadian workers looked at the outcome for secondary infertility after an ectopic pregnancy and found that in a study group of 70 such patients, 50 proceeded to investigation by hysteroscopy and laparoscopy, five of whom conceived, one had an ectopic pregnancy. The remaining 45 proceeded to laparoscopy at which 16 had irreparable tubes (length less than 4 cm, densely adherent adnexa, hydrosalpinx greater than 3 cm in diameter), 13 had no further surgery (four successful pregnancies and one ectopic), and 16 were considered for further surgery of whom two refused, three conceived while waiting for salpingolysis, five were still waiting for surgery, and, of six operated on, one delivered. Therefore in these 70 patients there were 13 live babies (18.6% pregnancy success rate) and 2 repeat ectopics (2.9%). These workers quoted Allan C. Barnes prophetic statement 'you should work as hard as possible to conserve the lady's tube in her first ectopic, just as you would if this were her second ectopic in her only remaining tube'.

Using microsurgical principles in cases of unruptured tubal ectopic pregnancy, it should be possible to evacuate the pregnancy with minimal tubal damage and at a later time when reactive oedema has subsided, carry out formal microsurgical tubal reconstruction (Winston 1978).

The most contemporary addition to microsurgery in gynaecology is the use of laser. At the 23rd British Congress of Obstetrics and Gynaecology in Birmingham in July 1983 Bellina from New Orleans presented an impressive series of some 200 infertile women in whom, following the use of microsurgery and laser, a pregnancy rate of more than 60% was achieved. Kelly & Roberts (1983) have used laser for neosalpingostomy, tubal reanastomosis, vaporization of adhesions, removal of endometriomatous deposits, removal of fibroids, and for metroplasty. They have not encountered any laser-induced complications and describe the main advantages of laser as decreased destruction of tissue, excellent haemostasis, precision of dissection and ablation, and shortened operating time—all important factors in the surgical management of endometriosis. The main disadvantage of laser according to Baggish (1983), apart from the capital cost of the equipment, was thermal damage consequent on heat production in target tissues by the laser beam. However, by varying the power density of the laser beam (a function of destructive spot size in millimetres and power output in watts) and the exposure time, it is possible to finesse out endometriomata even from precarious locations by using a long handled polished steel or titanium mirror to reflect the laser beam onto the target location. Chong & Baggish (1984) reported a 60.8% pregnancy success rate in a small group of 23 patients in whom CO_2 laser surgery was utilized and demonstrated the technique used in conservative procedures (adhesiolysis, wedge resection, vaporization of endometriomata etc.).

Several papers were presented to the April 1984 meeting of the American Fertility Society concerning the use of laser in gynaecology. The use with laparoscopy has already been mentioned. Comparing the outcome in terms of tubal patency rates using orthodox microsurgery or laser, McLaughlin (1984) and Diamond et al (1984) found improved patency rates after the use of laser.

In an experimental setting, Keye et al (1983) have used an argon laser on induced endometriosis in New Zealand rabbits. Using a 2 mm spot size and 2 W of power for 3–5 s exposure time, they found it was possible to ablate endometriosis completely with only 0.25 mm of thermal damage to underlying or surrounding tissues. These workers suggested that an argon laser could be advantageous in the treatment of endometriosis because of its selective absorption of haemoglobin pigmented tissues, and the ability of such a laser to be transmitted through a flexible tube system.

Since July 1980 a Coherent 400 carbon dioxide laser has been available for use in the Brisbane series. A small selected group of patients have had microsurgical repair and reconstruction utilizing CO_2 laser. All had bilateral tubal occlusion, some were desperation cases seen after repeated, failed attempts at IVF and ET, and overall these were patients for whom hopes of successful pregnancy looked dismal in the extreme. So far 12 patients have produced seven pregnancies in up to 2 years follow-up. There has been one ectopic pregnancy, one miscarriage in a patient who has subsequently had a successful term pregnancy, and four other full-term deliveries with one patient pregnant at the time of writing.

The major disadvantages in using this equipment are related to the cumbersome nature of the laser head of this particular unit and the need to manipulate the instrument, patient, and target area so that the destructive action of the laser used at reduced power output of 5–15 W can be utilized with microscopic precision to best advantage.

Since laparotomy and conservative surgery aim at preserving reproductive potential, what is the place of repeat laparotomy?

A series of 198 patients with endometriosis were evaluated by Schenken & Malinak (1978) over a 6-year period. Where indicated by diagnostic endoscopy, findings of endometriosis were staged according to the Acosta system, and laparotomy and conservative surgery were undertaken when no contraindications applied. Conservative treatment was the only method of treating endometriosis in these patients and included presacral neurectomy, sharp resection of endometriotic implants, lysis of adhesions, ventrosuspension of retroverted uteri and plication of the utero-sacral ligaments to improve uterine position.

A subgroup of patients requiring reoperation had been followed-up for at least 3 years after the first operation and 1 year after the second operation. While all but one in the subgroup for reoperation were infertile, the major indication for reoperation was painful disease. A total of 166 of their 198 patients had conservative surgery and 153 were infertile. The pregnancy rates in those patients with endometriosis alone, and no other infertility factors, after conservative surgery were 60% for mild, 50% for moderate, 25% for severe disease.

Subsequently 28 patients who had primary conservative surgery had a second operation for endometriosis. Two had a pelvic clearance, and, of the remaining 26 who had conservative surgery, nine had unilateral adnexectomy because of adhesive disease and destruction. Of these 26, 25 attempted pregnancy for at least one year after their second operation and only three conceived while three others subsequently required pelvic clearance for recurrent symptomatic endometriosis.

Of the 53 patients who became pregnant after the initial conservative operation, only two required reoperation—one with moderate and the other with severe disease. Sixty-four patients did not conceive after the first operation and 26 of these became the reoperation group discussed above.

Schenken & Malinak also found that two-thirds of their endometriosis patients had other infertility factors and reported excellent results when clomiphene citrate was used in those whose infertility was related to anovulation and endometriosis, a result in agreement with the Brisbane series findings. These authors found the average time lapse to second operation was 14.4 months for mild, 32.8 months for moderate, and 31.9 months for severe endometriosis. However, in terms of fertility after reoperation only a disappointing three of 25 infertile patients conceived after second operation.

On the face of it these results might not seem encouraging, and while these workers raise the important issue of coincidental infertility factors—an issue that bedevils attempts to assess the results of treatment in 'pure' and 'complicated' endometriosis—reoperation in the absence of contraindications should be available for those patients wishing to retain their fertility potential despite the insidious progression of endometriosis not yet to stage IV level.

Radical surgery

Often the degree of disability produced by endometriosis is disproportionate to the extent or stage of the disease (Counseller 1949). Accordingly the extent of surgery offered to an endometriosis sufferer will vary according to her age, her fertility needs, and the amount of disability experienced as well as her wishes in the matter and the stage of the disease.

The traditional notion that radical surgery in endometriosis invariably involved removal of both ovaries has been successfully challenged by several authors. Smith (1978) stated that hysterectomy with excision of all endometriotic tissue is the most effective surgical treatment for endometriosis in women at, or near, 40 years of age with extensive disease. To achieve relief from symptoms prior to the menopause, it is not automatically necessary to remove both ovaries. The conservation of healthy, normal ovarian tissue at hysterectomy in such patients, as will be shown shortly, is quite justifiable (Fig. 6.1).

Where bilateral oophorectomy is performed as part of the surgical cure, the problem arises as to how to manage post-castration symptoms in the premenopausal patient. Supportive hormonal replacement medication and emotional support therapy will be needed if the ovaries are sacrificed. Some women can be curiously vicious to their own kind and frequently seem to delight in maliciously destroying—often under the guise of helpful concern— the tattered remnants of self-esteem and self confidence held by those in whom bilateral oophorectomy was necessary. Joel-Cohen (1978) in discussing hysterectomy mentions the importance of communication and explanation to patients of what is intended surgically, and what actually happens in reality at operation. The author has, for many years, used the educational leaflets on hysterectomy produced by the Queensland Health Education Council (Fig. 6.2a, b) for the purpose of explanation and uses these to reinforce the view that radical surgery is not synonymous with being condemned to a bleak future—fat, hirsute, sexless.

The emotional aspects of hysterectomy and the post-hysterectomy depression syndrome were considered in detail by Sloan (1978) and he identified several important factors in relation to feminine function and sexuality after hysterectomy—mainly loss of status associated with the feminine mystique, loss of the security of having an intact body with intact genitalia, and loss of acceptance as a woman—be it threatened, symbolic or real. He also found that the ability to menstruate was seen as a credit, not a debit, point by a majority of women, and that the effect of the stress of surgery was probably not truly appreciated by surgeons in considering post-hysterectomy depression.

Richards (1978) on the subject of hysterectomy proposed three categories of indications for hysterectomy.

1. Life threatening or health threatening indications
2. Patient indicated hysterectomy for disability and quality of life considerations
3. Prophylactic hysterectomy

In a series of 340 hysterectomies he showed an incidence of 80 in category 1, 253 in category 2, and seven in category 3. Most patients having radical surgery in the Brisbane series are Richards' category 2 cases. Richards preoperatively discussed with his patients the mortality rate (16.4 per 10 000) of hysterectomy and major complications such as fistula, thromboembolism etc. then, as happened in the Brisbane series, left category 2 patients to decide when they wanted radical surgery performed.

The other somewhat irrelevant, but important, issue mentioned in Richards' paper, is the fact that there were more patients requiring hysterectomy following vasectomy in male partners, than tubal ligation in female patients—also a common experience in the Brisbane practice.

Endometriosis often presents the gynaecological surgeon with situations as challenging as one could meet in pelvic surgery and both Smith (1978) and Pratt & Williams (1980) emphasized the importance in extensive disease of first restoring anatomical normality before proceeding to resection, if surgical damage to bowel and bladder are to be minimized. Pratt & Williams believed that proper surgical training of the gynaecologist is important if the patient is to receive the best possible surgical help in endometriosis of major degree. Their approach to radical surgery is orthodox and they only advocate 'unroofing' the ureters if the disease process makes their course in the pelvis difficult to identify visually, or by palpation. They believe that surgeons should be prepared for all surgical eventualities (e.g. bowel resection if indicated) in radical operations for endometriosis and, certainly in stage IV disease, intravenous urography and suitable bowel preparation are most useful prerequisites prior to radical surgery. While Smith found sympathy for those surgeons who find themselves obliged to perform a sub-total hysterectomy because of technical difficulties, Joel-Cohen

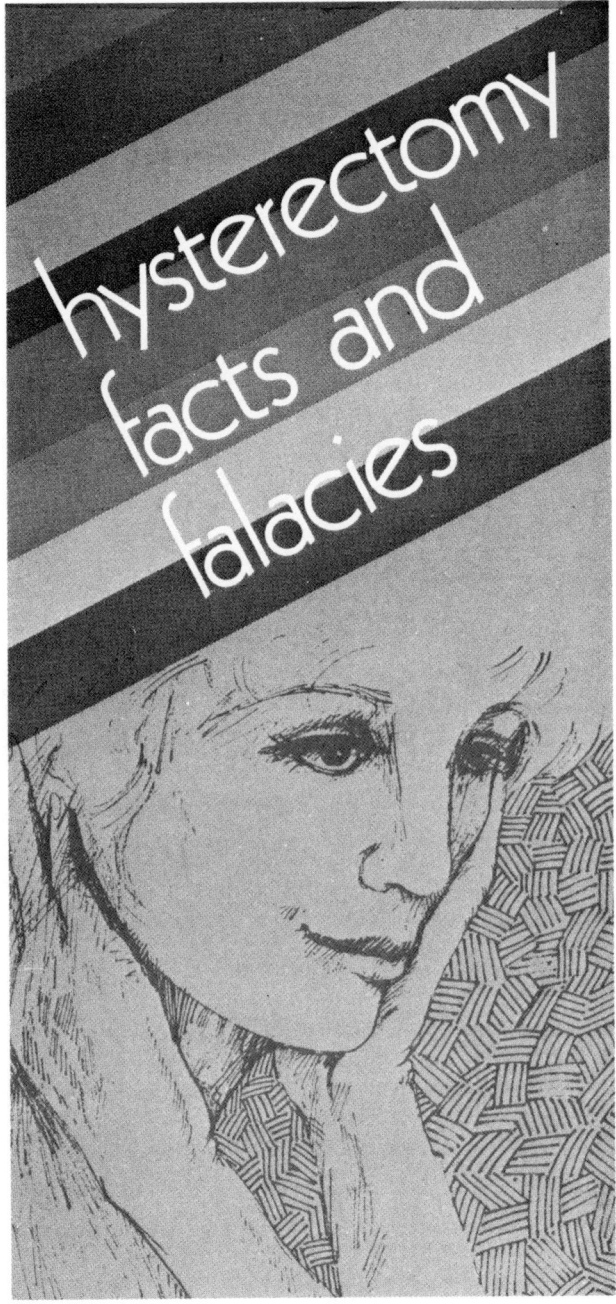

Fig. 6.2(a) Educational leaflet on hysterectomy, produced by the Queensland Health Education Council

WHAT MAKES THE OPERATION NECESSARY?

In the past, hysterectomy was sometimes used to cure complaints which now can often be treated successfully with drugs, for example in cases of heavy bleeding.

Ancient Greeks believed that a woman's emotions were made in her womb, for which the Greek name was "hysteros". From this origin came the word, "hysterical". Of course it has long been known that emotions originate in the brain — but if the emotion — whether it is due to anxiety, frustration or unhappiness — remains for long enough, it can cause heavy periods. At one time the only known remedy was hysterectomy, which cured the heavy periods, but left the disturbed emotions unaltered. Now drugs and a sympathetic understanding of the problem usually are adequate to deal with the condition.

However, there are some conditions for which the only successful answer is hysterectomy.

Apart from such obvious reasons as cancer of the uterus or cervix, muscle tumours, or "fibroids" are the most common conditions for which a hysterectomy is the only really complete answer.

Fibroids begin with the overdevelopment of one or more of the muscle fibres which make up the wall of the uterus. They grow into pea-sized tumours deep in the muscle wall, and continue to grow slowly until they reach the size of a golf ball, a tennis ball or even a grapefruit. They may be few or many and can grow outward or inward. If they grow inward and distort the shape of the uterine cavity, menstrual periods may be heavy or irregular.

In rare cases, fibroids can cause pain during sexual intercourse. The medical terms for this painful coitus is dyspareunia.

Other frequent indications for hysterectomy are "adenomyosis" and the related "endometriosis" both non-malignant disturbances of the glandular uterine lining.

WILL THE OVARIES BE REMOVED?

No doctor will remove a woman's ovaries before her menopause unless it is absolutely essential. Sometimes it is necessary to remove one ovary, but if both are diseased, every effort will be made to leave some ovarian tissue to carry on its work of producing the female sex hormone oestrogen, if the disease is non-cancerous.

If it is necessary to remove both ovaries and the patient is not past the menopause, the gynaecologist will make sure his patient is given oestrogen tablets to replace the hormone and minimise "change of life" symptoms which would otherwise follow the operation. In certain cases of cancer however oestrogen is not used.

THE EFFECT OF HYSTERECTOMY.

The after-effects of hysterectomy will be that menstruation ceases, and that pregnancy cannot possibly occur.

Hysterectomy, or removal of the womb, is one of the most common surgical operations performed on women. Unfortunately, it is also one of the most maligned by those who do not understand it.

questions you may ask . . .

Q. Will hysterectomy affect my sex life?

A. No. Hysterectomy does not make a woman sexually mutilated and undesirable; it does not shorten her vagina so that sexual intercourse is impossible or potentially dangerous. In most cases, when the womb is removed, the vagina is cut at its uppermost end, and the cervix no longer projects into it, so if anything, the vagina is a little longer after the operation. In rare cases, the cervix is left when the surgeon removes the section of the womb above it. In such a case, there is no alteration at all to the vagina.

Q. Must I take some medication for the rest of my life?

A. No, unless both ovaries are removed. Then you will need to take only the oestrogen tablets, to replace natural hormones — and these only for a limited time.

Q. Will I suffer a personality change?

A. This is really up to you. If you convince yourself you will be changed nothing will prevent you from becoming a chronic neurotic. But the operation will not cause it!

Q. How soon will I be able to return to normal duties?

A. As with any other major surgery, it is advisable to "take things quietly" for a few weeks, and gradually increase activity rather than rush into it. Your doctor will advise about the length of time needed for convalescence — usually six weeks.

Q. Will I be a semi-invalid for the rest of my life?

A. No. You will no doubt feel healthier than before the operation, as the complaint for which it has been advised will be cured.

Q. Would an outsider know I had had a hysterectomy?

A. There will be no visible signs. Many of the women you pass daily in the street, or work with, have had the same kind of operation.

If you or your husband have any further questions, or fears you would like to allay, talk it over with your doctor. He — not an uninformed relative or friend — is qualified to advise.

Q. But will sex be as satisfying to me after the operation?

A. There will be no difference in sexual desire or satisfaction **after** the hysterectomy. In fact, where there has been some fear of pregnancy, when all possibility of pregnancy has been removed, a woman's sexual desires and reponse may increase.

Q. Will I still be able to reach an orgasm, or "climax" during intercourse?

A. Yes. Removal of the womb has no effect on this.

Q. Will my husband be able to feel any physical change in my body, when we have sexual intercourse?

A. No. Unless he was told, a man would not know a woman had undergone this type of surgery.

Q. How soon after the operation should my husband and I resume normal sexual relations?

A. Once the top of the vagina has healed strongly, which takes about six weeks, sexual intercourse can be resumed safely and with normal satisfaction.

Q. Will I become fat?

A. Only if you sit about and eat too much instead of carrying on normal activities. Women who grow fat after any surgery, usually do so because during convalescence a pattern of over-eating and under-exercising is set, and this begins a habit difficult to break.

Q. Will I become hairy or develop male characteristics?

A. No. The womb does not produce any hormones — the ovaries do this — so removal of the womb will make no difference to hormone balance.

Q. Will I go through an immediate "change of life"?

A. Only if both ovaries are completely removed, in which case the oestrogen tablets you will be given, will minimise or completely relieve, symptoms.

Division of Health Education & Information,
Queensland Health Department,
5-9 Costin Street, Fortitude Valley.
P.O. Box 155, Fortitude Valley 4006.

(1978) was more critical of the sub-total operation, probably because he had seen 14 cases of cervical stump cancer in his career.

Some American series report the use of presacral neurectomy in the treatment of endometriosis (Buttram 1979b), Polan & de Cherney 1980) and pelvic pain, but others (Sadigh et al 1977) have not resorted to this procedure which was not employed in the Brisbane series.

Radical surgery in endometriosis must always be performed by the abdominal route. Even if the pouch of Douglas and utero-vesical fold are not distorted by disease, the limited visual access through the vaginal vault renders it impossible to resect all endometriomata to the extent that is possible through an abdominal incision. There

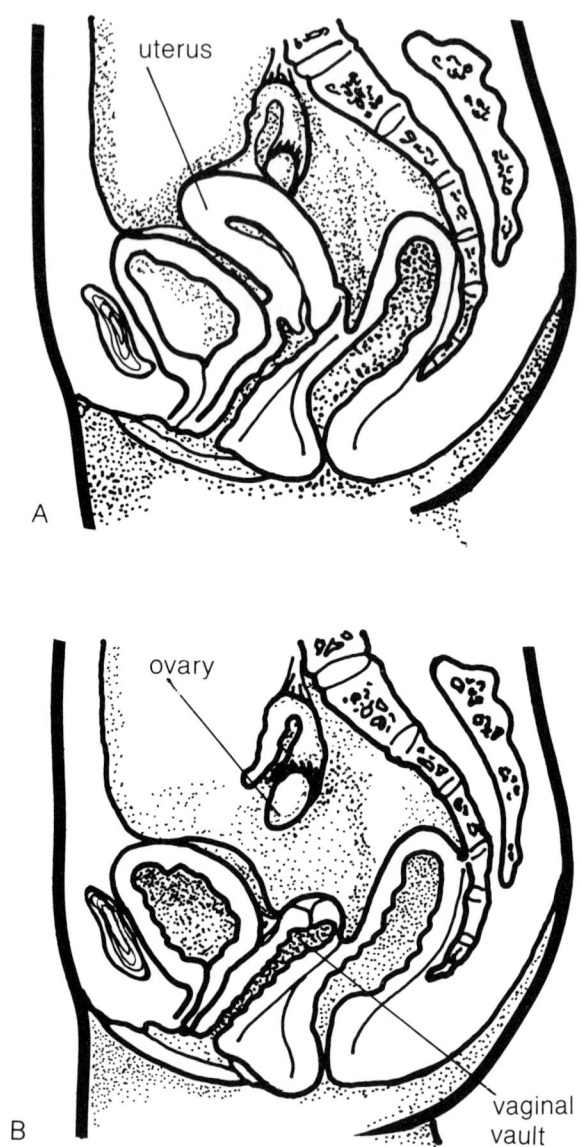

The length of the vagina shown in A is not shortened by hysterectomy shown in B.

Fig. 6.2(b) Diagram taken from educational leaflet produced by the Queensland Health Education Council showing that the vagina is not shortened by hysterectomy

are of course occasions, fortunately rare, when a combined approach is necessary to remove extra-vaginal endometriomata.

There is often a considerable bare area left on the pelvic peritoneum after resection and clearance of all endometriomata. The decision to reperitonealize with a peritoneal or omental graft, to leave the vaginal vault open to allow free drainage of ongoing vascular and lymphatic ooze, or to close the vault and drain the pelvic cavity transabdominally with a sump drain and continuous low pressure suction, and the role of prophylactic antibiotics, and techniques of abdominal wall closure in the face of certain postoperative ileus after a radical resection of endometriosis, are all matters of personal judgement by the surgeon.

Certain axioms, however, hold true:

1. Endometriotic tissue is always in danger of becoming necrotic and infected
2. Bowel involvement and resection may lead to faecal contamination even in the most experienced surgical hands
3. Any disease that produces anatomic distortion in the pelvis will pose a surgical threat to the ureters in the pelvis
4. When confronted with overwhelming surgical problems appropriately expert help should be sought and the author is grateful to John Herron, general surgeon, and John Phillips, urological surgeon, for their assistance with the most difficult stage IV cases in the Brisbane series

One of the major problems in the private practice situation in Brisbane is that a gynaecologist often operates with a general practitioner assistant, usually the practitioner who has referred the patient initially. This is obviously good practice, ethical, good public relations, and a mutually amicable arrangement. However, when trouble looms, the surgeon is then in a predicament and it takes great courage to acknowledge, with possible loss of face in the presence of the referring general practitioner, that more expert assistance is required than he is capable of offering. As in all surgical matters, operative skill and the patient's needs must override all other considerations.

Results of surgical treatment

All 717 patients in the Bribane series had at least one surgical operation, where the diagnosis was made and the disease process was staged. The results of this primary surgery are shown in Table 6.1. Relevant factors considered were stage of disease, type of operation, apparent cure (either clinically free of disease, or pregnancy in the case of those who were infertile), or persistent clinical features of disease. If having been classified as cured, the patient re-presented with new clinical features or new operative findings of endometriosis such an event was recorded as a recurrence.

Table 6.1 Results after primary surgery for the Brisbane series

Stage	0	1	2	3	4	Totals
Total cases	18	241	254	165	39	717
Conservative surgery						
Laparoscopy	17	196	159	40	2	414
Laparotomy	1	19	36	47	8	111
Hysterectomy		17	33	47	7 ⎱	168
Hysterectomy + BSO			12	30	22 ⎰	
Other operation		9	14	1		24
Cure	11	79	106	88	25	309
Persistent disease	4	37	47	33	6	127
Recurrent disease	2	63	66	17	4	152
Lost to follow-up	1	62	35	27	4	129

BSO: bilateral salpingo-oophorectomy

The 'lost to follow-up' group includes many patients who live too remotely from Brisbane for follow-up (e.g. New Guinea, Vanuatu, Christmas Island in the Indian Ocean, Kingdom of Tonga, and remote areas of Queensland up to 1200 miles from Brisbane). Others are patients dissatisfied with either the service provided or the results of side-effects of treatment offered, who, as is their right, sought help elsewhere.

A quick scan of Table 6.1 suggests that the cure rate for less severe stages of endometriosis is appallingly bad. However, it will also be noted from this table that the progression and extent of the surgical attack increases with the stage of disease and with the more severe stages radical operations were more common and obviously more likely to be curative. Conversely, more patients in the lesser stages of endometriosis had multiple coexistent disease entities associated with endometriosis and, of course, more were left with potential reproductive function for longer than those having radical surgery, thus increasing the likelihood of a recurrence.

Several patients with extensive disease have refused possible curative radical surgery. There are six patients with stage 3 disease presently on continuous progestogen therapy who have deferred major surgery until a more convenient time, a further 28 stage 3 patients are continuing with continuous progestogen therapy long-term because they hope, in the future, to attempt conception. This same hope applies to two of the stage 4 patients who have refused to consider radical ablative surgery. Nine of these 30 stage 3 and 4 patients are as yet unmarried and not in steady relationships but wish to preserve their fertility options.

Patients treated by laparotomy had coincidental diseases treated surgically as follows: myomectomy 14; unilateral ovarian cystectomy 26; bilateral ovarian cystectomy 13; ventrosuspension 26; judicious debulking of peritoneal lesions 63; excision of fulguration of bowel or bladder lesions 31.

Where primary peritoneal closure was not possible after extensive peritoneal stripping procedures, peritoneal grafts using anterolateral parietal flaps have been used on nine occasions with good results.

The incidence of coincidental disease (polycystic ovary disease, pelvic inflammatory disease, etc.) in patients with less severe forms of endometriosis also contributed to the poor results of primary treatment, not just in terms of failure to cure with successful pregnancy when the complaint was infertility, but also in terms of persistent symptoms or signs (e.g. where the original symptom was dysmenorrhoea or menstrual irregularity, the computer was unable to distinguish the subtleties necessary to determine whether endometriosis or one of the coincidental disease problems, such as pelvic inflammatory disease, had produced the symptoms or signs recorded).

Those patients having hysterectomy without bilateral adnexec-tomy represent a personal viewpoint concerning radical surgery in endometriosis and reflect a deliberate policy as opposed to surgical carelessness. Contemporary premenopausal women in Brisbane will not lightly accept offers of surgical castration, especially if this means removing healthy ovaries, even after explanation of the mechanisms of cure of endometriosis anticipated, following bilateral oophorec-tomy. The experience with post-hysterectomy progestogens in the Brisbane series suggests this is a reasonable position to take. In the case of depot medroxyprogesterone acetate in particular, a long-term disease-free status may possibly be maintained without the need for secondary surgery. It is also possible that the use of gonadotrophin-releasing hormone agonists to produce a medical oophorectomy may help solve the surgeon's dilemma over this issue of ovarian preservation in the future.

Of those patients having obligatory bilateral salpingo-oophorec-tomy not only on theoretical grounds, but also on realistic grounds, such as bilateral adnexal disease (39 of 64), 47 have received injections of depot medroxyprogesterone acetate 150 mg/ml at 3-monthly intervals for up to 4 years postoperatively in order to prevent the onset of castration symptoms, to block the activity of any microscopic deposits of endometriosis inadvertently left behind at surgery, and to prevent further endometriosis from developing. This programme has been most successful in 44 patients and the only problem now is when to stop therapy. A minimum of 12 months of such therapy seems sensible.

Primary surgery without fertility preservation

There were 320 patients in the Brisbane series who, following primary surgery, had lost their potential fertility. They had either a hysterectomy, a bilateral tubal occlusion for sterilization, or bilateral adnexectomy prior to, or during, primary surgery. Ninety-seven of these patients were lost to follow-up by the end of a 12-month period. Of the remaining 223, 149 (67%) were regarded as cured while 49 (22%) had residual persisting symptoms or signs for which they received medical therapy, and 25 (11%) had recurrent disease, surgically proven. This latter group includes mostly patients from the early days when diagnostic laparoscopy only was combined with pseudopregnancy using combination oral contraceptives—a programme so useless as to be now totally abandoned. Two patients in this group suffered unwanted ectopic pregnancies following unipolar bilateral tubal diathermy for sterilization at the time of laparoscopy.

Primary surgery with preservation of fertility— pregnancy outcome

Following primary surgery, or previous surgery, 397 of the 717 patients in the Brisbane series had retained their reproductive potential. Of these, 221 wished to conceive and 140 were successful, producing 441 pregnancies in all during the years from February 1967 to December 1983—a conception rate of 63%.

It must be emphasized that the number of total pregnancies was not only limited by gynaecological factors, but by the patients' wishes based on socio-economic and other factors. During the years of the study the average family size in Brisbane declined dramatically under the influence of the zero population growth philosophy, the economic necessity of mothers to return to work, and the legitimate emotional and intellectual needs of many women to pursue a career outside the home, in addition to, or instead of, mothering. Ethnic needs varied also. The high parity of Tongan women, while traditionally prized in that community, would be unacceptable to the majority of Brisbane women. So reproductive potential was not open ended and the figure of 441 conceptions may have been limited by these other considerations and not be a true reflection of the real unlimited potential fertility of these women.

Of the 441 post-therapy pregnancies 367 were successful and produced 367 live children. There were two sets of twins in clomiphene-induced pregnancies in mothers with coincidental polycystic ovary disease. Two stillbirths resulted from cord complications after week 32 of pregnancy; 66 spontaneous abortions occurred (15% of conceptions) and one patient had a termination of pregnancy performed elsewhere, while seven suffered tubal ectopic pregnancies. Three of these seven ectopic pregnancies occurred after previous microsurgical adnexal reconstruction for endometriosis with coincidental pelvic inflammatory disease. This incidence of ectopic pregnancy of one in 60 conceptions is higher than the one in 150 conceptions noted prior to treatment and is in keeping with the experience of Wheeler & Malinak (1983).

Recurrent disease

After a minimum follow-up of 12 months, 152 patients had recurrent disease and 127 patients had persistent symptoms (including infertility), signs, or both, of endometriosis. Of these 279 women 245 then had further surgery as shown in Table 6.2. After conservative surgery as a second surgical procedure, of 176 women wishing to conceive (83 of whom were still nulliparous) 75 subsequently had

Table 6.2 Second operation—type of operation performed

Laparoscopy	57	
Laparotomy		
unilateral ovarian cystectomy	39 ⎤	
bilateral ovarian cystectomy	24 ⎬ 119	
unilateral adnexectomy	41 ⎟	
laser therapy	15 ⎦	
Hysterectomy	49 ⎤ 69	
Hysterectomy + BSO	20 ⎦	

BSO: bilateral salpingo-oophorectomy

babies—36 from the nulliparous group. This is a very satisfactory pregnancy rate of 43% in keeping with the most recent findings of Wheeler et al (1983).

Third operation for recurrent disease

Further surgery was carried out for recurrent disease in 32 patients (Table 6.3) of whom seven had pregnancies, three with surviving babies.

Table 6.3 Third operation—type of operation performed

Laparoscopy	10	
Laparotomy		
unilateral ovarian cystectomy	4 ⎫	
bilateral ovarian cystectomy	2 ⎬	7
laser ablation and salpingostomy	1 ⎭	
TAH + progestins	11 ⎫	15
TAH + BSO	4 ⎭	

TAH: total abdominal hysterectomy
BSO: bilateral salpingo-oophorectomy

Fourth operation for recurrent disease

Two patients in the Brisbane series have had four operations. Both had pelvic clearances for intractable symptoms—one patient had sadly managed an ectopic pregnancy and two miscarriages from her multiple attempts at successful conception, while the other has two surviving children from three successful pregnancies.

Relationship of successful pregnancy to subsequent recurrent disease

The results of the Brisbane series offer no reason to challenge the statement of McArthur & Ulfelder (1965) that:

1. Endometriosis behaves extremely variably in pregnancy
2. There is a decreased tissue responsiveness to hormonal stimulation, rather than a necrosis of lesions, which leads to regression of endometriosis in pregnancy
3. Following pregnancy, persistent disease is encountered more often than permanent cure.

Of the 140 patients who conceived after primary treatment and were still available for follow-up, 84 had surgically diagnosed recurrent disease between 1 and 12 years after confinement—a recurrence rate of 60%. The majority of these recurrences occurred between 1 and 4 years after confinement. Of the 146 patients with successful conceptions, 67 had lactated for a minimum of 6 months, 29 for 9 months, and five for 12 months or longer so lactational amenorrhoea does not seem to confer any consistent preventative benefit in terms of recurrent endometriosis.

Secondary surgical treatment produced 22 successful conceptions in the 55 parous patients who attempted pregnancy. Twenty-nine patients of the 84 with recurrent disease opted to cease trying for pregnancy following previous success. Of the 22 successful second conceptions following treatment, 19 surviving babies including one set of twins were delivered, a second set of twins aborted at 16 weeks' gestation because of an unsuspected incompetent cervix, and two of the other patients aborted, while one had an ectopic pregnancy following extensive laser microsurgical repair and reconstruction for endometriosis and pelvic inflammatory disease.

Seven of those who successfully conceived after second surgery subsequently were demonstrated surgically to have a further recurrence of endometriosis requiring a third surgical attack. Four of these patients conceived and three had surviving babies while one had an ectopic pregnancy. Unfortunately this was this patient's second ectopic pregnancy. The two patients having fourth operations have been previously mentioned.

Since the data collection for the Brisbane series stopped in January 1983, a successful in vitro fertilization and embryo transfer programme has been established in Brisbane and where pregnancy is desired, the need to operate and reoperate, as in the past in this series, will hopefully be reduced and patients will achieve pregnancy with the aid of this new high technology programme without running the risks of repeated surgical attacks. Although the results in this Brisbane series are already good and equal to those obtained elsewhere, the overall pregnancy success rate of 20–25% (Craft 1984) achieved world-wide will hopefully be considerably improved.

While there were no cases of acute surgical crisis in pregnancy due to endometriosis complications such as the ruptured endometrioma reported by Rossman et al (1983), one patient who had a Caesarean section performed for a clinical diagnosis of acute abdominal pain due to an accidental haemorrhage at 37 weeks also had a 3 cm infarcted ovarian endometrioma.

Preconception drug therapy

Following primary surgery, especially where this was limited to laparoscopic surgery, drug therapy, as suggested by Kistner (1975), was used before patients attempted conception.

Table 6.4 shows the distribution of drug therapy in the 221 patients attempting conception. It will be noted that there were 16 cases of minimal disease and no coincidental pathology where no drug therapy was used, and 11 of these patients were pregnant within 12 months of primary surgery (69%), in keeping with the findings of Puolakka et al (1980).

Table 6.4 Preconception drug therapy—drugs used

	No.	Pregnancy
Norethisterone	77	51
Medroxyprogesterone	45	29
Clomiphene	55	42 (twins × 2)
Dydrogesterone	8	3
Danazol	20	4
No drug therapy	16	11
Total	221	140

The pregnancy rate in 77 patients who were given norethisterone subsequent to primary surgery was 66%, after medroxyprogesterone acetate 64%, after danazol 20%, and after dydrogesterone 38%.

Clomiphene produced a 76% pregnancy rate and was used in patients with coincidental polycystic ovary disease and luteinizing unruptured follicle syndrome (43), of whom 11 also had pelvic inflammatory disease and three had fibroids.

The other 12 patients receiving clomiphene included a small group whose husbands worked at a remote distance from home where, because conception opportunities were limited, clomiphene was used judiciously to facilitate conception opportunity during infrequent coital encounters. Danazol will be considered in depth later.

Complications of surgery

Laparoscopy

There were no significant complications in the Brisbane series in the 481 laparoscopic operations apart from the two undesired ectopic pregnancies that followed coincident bilateral, unipolar tubal diathermy for sterilization at the time of treating endometriosis.

Laparotomy

There were 237 laparotomies performed in all and the highest incidence of complications occurred, sadly, in this group where obviously, in the interests of preservation of fertility potential it was of prime importance to have fewest complications. The problems encountered were:

1. Paralytic ileus—5 cases
2. Adhesive bowel obstruction requiring surgical relief—3 cases
3. Infected wound haematoma—2 cases
4. Pelvic abscess—1 case
5. Pulmonary embolus—1 case

Myomectomy and adnexal reconstruction figured prominently in the patients having postoperative bowel problems and it is possible that the difficulty in securing haemostasis at myomectomy is reflected in the higher incidence of haemorrhage-induced bowel complications.

Hysterectomy

A total of 254 hysterectomies were performed and the only significant complications were:

1. Paralytic ileus—3 cases
2. Retroperitoneal ureteric obstruction by haematoma requiring evacuation—1 case
3. Ureteric stenosis by extraperitoneal scar tissue 1 month postoperatively—1 case
4. Wound haematoma requiring evacuation—1 case

In the last few years the use of wound drainage has been extended so that it is virtually a routine procedure and wound complications have diminished enormously.

There have been no deaths associated with endometriosis or its treatment in this series, although one young patient has died as the result of an accidental electrocution, and another patient died of metastases from primary carcinoma of a retained fallopian tube, associated with retention, at her request, of an apparently healthy tube and ovary at hysterectomy and unilateral adnexectomy performed for recurrent stage 2 disease prior to the menopause. The tubal tumour presented with bladder pressure symptoms nearly 2 years after hysterectomy. This patient was not given post-hysterectomy progestins.

Medical treatment of endometriosis

A variety of suggested non-surgical methods for curing or controlling endometriosis has been hailed with enthusiasm and hope over the last 25 years. First the replacement of the then existing oestrogen or androgen treatment programmes with the 'pseudopregnancy' programme first mentioned by Kistner in 1958; then 'pseudomenopause' therapy utilizing danazol was hailed with fulsome praise after Greenblatt et al (1971) published the first report of this preparation and its clinical uses. More recently 'medical oophorectomy' therapy using gonadotrophin-releasing hormone agonists has been reported as showing promising results in treating patients with endometriosis. The frustrating truism about all available medical treatment programmes developed so far, is that there is no preparation which is totally free from side-effects and 100% effective in all patients, available to treat endometriosis at present.

Pseudopregnancy therapy

In 1958 Kistner published a paper entitled 'The use of newer progestins in the treatment of endometriosis' wherein he reported the results of treating 12 patients with clinically diagnosed endometriosis with large doses of oestrogen and progestogen in a graduated fashion over 7 months, as an alternative to pregnancy-induced improvement in endometriosis. Kistner used the expression 'pseudopregnancy' to describe the biological changes he had induced in these patients. He was subsequently taken to task by Beecham in a letter to the Editor of the *American Journal of Obstetrics and Gynecology* in July 1958 for not giving credit for this concept to both Joe Meigs, who had expounded his views on a possible aetiological factor in endometriosis in 1938 and possible alleviation of endometriosis in 1949, and to Karnaky (1948) who, Beecham (1958) felt, had produced a drug-induced amenorrhoea state with stilboestrol, thus using a pseudopregnancy form of treatment. In reply to this letter Kistner pointed out that he did not regard the use of diethylstilboestrol alone as inducing a 'pseudopregnancy' state, a term which he said had been previously used by many authors (Bradbury J J, Brown W, Rock J, and Horne H W) to indicate a state induced by the simultaneous prolonged use of oestrogens and progesterones.

Notwithstanding these slight historical diversions, Kistner's name has, since 1958, been associated with the concept of producing a hyperhormonal pseudopregnancy state to alleviate the clinical features of endometriosis. The drugs he used initially were diethylstilboestrol or ethinyloestradiol and 17α-hydroxyprogesterone caproate, and norethynodrel which, when used with 1.5% ethinyloeastradiol in tablet form, was available as one of the early contraceptive pills marketed under the trade name Enovid.

Noting that Meigs had advocated early marriage and early childbearing as prophylactic measures to avoid the development of endometriosis, Kistner more reasonably pointed out that this was not an option available to everybody and that there was a definite need to try to produce the biological advantages of a pregnancy state without the inappropriate production of a baby. He was very encouraged by his results in the first 12 patients whose outcome he reported, and he noted that the only side-effects occurred in the patients who were taking up to 40 mg of Enovid daily or had received up to 500 mg of 17α-hydroxyprogesterone caproate weekly, when nausea without vomiting, and breast soreness were noted. Kistner noted physical improvement after 3–4 months of therapy in the endometriotic state and was able, in one patient, to demonstrate decidual changes in endometriosis deposits.

The progestins used were thought to be safe and free from side-effects. Hydroxyprogesterone followed a different metabolic pathway to free progesterone which produced increased pregnandiol excretion in urine as its metabolic end product. The use of hydroxyprogesterone caproate showed a reduction in pregnandiol excretion as seen in ovulation inhibition, and it was believed that most of the esterified steroid was transported intact to the tissues where it exerted its biological activity, and, at the same time, was metabolized slowly. Norethynodrel has been demonstrated in animal experiments to have a potent progesterone-like activity when administered orally and was thought to be free from androgenic or cortisone-like side-effects. It was of low toxicity and it was believed to suppress gonadotrophin secretion.

It was on the basis that pregnancy was believed to have a benign effect on endometriosis due to the decidual reaction created in endometriotic lesions with areas of necrosis following this activity, and the belief that this was directly related to the increased levels of oestrogen and progesterone produced endogenously in pregnancy that Kistner and subsequent developers of the notion of this form of hormone therapy for endometriosis pursued their therapeutic goals. As more oral contraceptive preparations came on the market with combinations of either ethinyloestradiol or mestranol as oestrogenic compounds together with a variety of progestogenic compounds (l-norgestrel, d-l-norgestrel, norethisterone, norethisterone acetate, ethynodiol diacetate, lynoestrenol, medroxyprogesterone), the range of available preparations widened and when side-effects resulted in patient reluctance to comply with prescribing, it was an easy matter to change to a different hormonal combination. As a result, the treatment of endometriosis with an assortment of synthetic hormones became confusing and the comparative results virtually unassessable.

Progestogen pharmacology

As is seen from Figure 6.3 all progestational agents share a common steroidal four-ring nucleus and synthetic progestogens are derived either from progesterone or 19-nortestosterone. The commonly used agents in the Brisbane series were medroxyprogesterone acetate, norethisterone (norethindrone), and norethisterone acetate.

Unfortunately there has been considerable disagreement from one study to another about the reliability of relative progestogenic potencies on these assorted compounds. Qualitatively, bioassays have suggested medroxyprogesterone acetate, megestrol acetate, and D-norgestrel have strong progestational activity, while norethisterone and norethynodrel have relatively weak progestational activity.

Subcellular research mentioned by Brenner (1982) has disclosed that steroids passively diffuse across cell menbranes in both directions. At cellular level of the target organ the first step leading to an expression of steroid hormone action is the formation of a cytoplasm receptor-steroid complex. This binding of the steroid to its specific cytocell receptor is structurally specific. Structural changes then occur in the steroid-receptor complex allowing the transport of the complex into the nucleus. Within the nucleus the steroid-receptor complex is then bound to the chromatin. This step alters the production of messenger RNA which is transported to the cytoplasm where it effects cellular protein production resulting in an expression of steroid action by the target organ.

The ability of steroids to bind to specific receptors has led to the definition of a progestational agent as 'one that binds to the progesterone receptor' (Edgren 1980).

Progesterone receptor synthesis is influenced by both progesterone and oestrogen concentrations in the target issue. Oestrogen enhances the production of progestogen receptors and oestrogen receptors, while progesterone inhibits the production of both types of receptors.

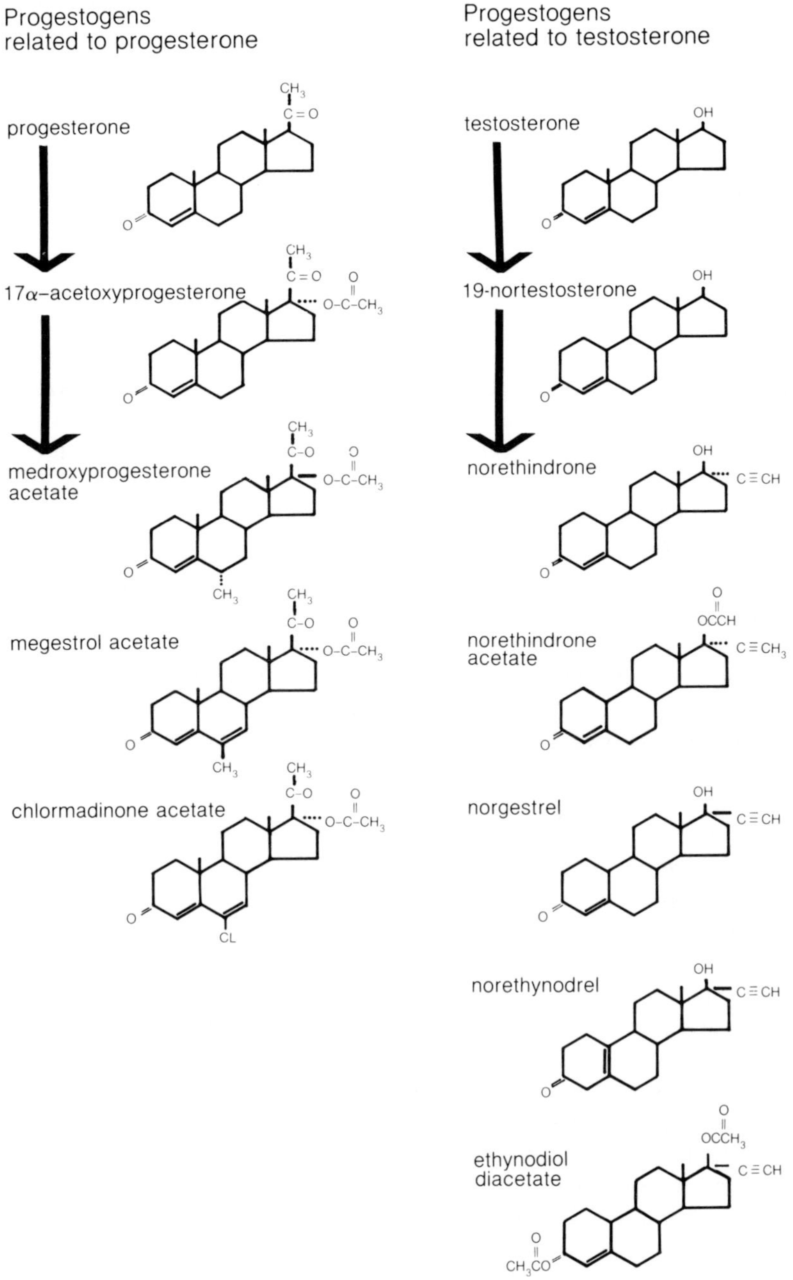

Fig. 6.3 Derivation of progestogens

In target tissue not previously stimulated by oestrogen, the concentration of progesterone receptors is very low and progesterone and synthetic progestogens have little biological activity in such tissues.

The human uterus primed with oestrogen contains high concentrations of progesterone receptors in both endometrium and myometrium; perhaps ectopically located endometrium in endometriosis has a similar concentration.

The affinity of progestational agents for the progesterone receptors in oestrogen-primed endometrium and myometrium can be used as the parameter for differentiating progestogenic activity in various compounds. The greater the potency of a compound, the greater will be the progesterone receptor binding. The progestogens l-norgestrel and norethisterone are bound more or less equally to progesterone receptors; medroxyprogesterone acetate is only a little less strongly bound.

Androgen activity generated by progestogens has always concerned clinicians. The relative androgenic activity of various progestational agents has been compared, in a biological situation, using a measure of the amount of radiolabelled steroid displaced by the test substance from androgen receptors in the rat prostate, or by bioassay of rat prostate growth stimulated by progestogenic agents. In both these techniques norethisterone was found to have far more androgenicity than medroxyprogesterone, but was not as potentially androgenic as D-l-norgestrel, l-norgestrel, or ethynodiol acetate.

The oestrogenic effect of progestogenic agents was assessed by studies measuring the displacement of radiolabelled oestradiol from the rabbit uterine cytocell receptors. These tests showed that norethisterone, norethynodrel and ethinyl diacetate have a weak affinity for oestrogen receptors but no displacement occurred with other progestogens. In the case of norethisterone it is thought that the weak oestrogenic activity is not due so much to conversion to an oestrogenic substance but rather by competition with oestrogen for oestrogen receptors, or by the inhibition of synthesis of oestrogen receptors (Clark et al 1977).

The anti-oestrogenic activity of these progestational agents has important clinical application in all branches of female biology and medical practice. It is generally accepted that the addition of a little progesterone to oestrogen replacement therapy, where indicated, will reduce the likelihood of the development of neoplastic changes in endometrium and breast tissue. The progestogens decrease the

116

synthesis of oestrogen receptors thereby reducing the risk of the development of cancer in these organs.

Atherogenicity of sex steroids

At a biochemical level an important practical consideration is the effect of ingested steroid hormones on plasma lipids and the link with atherosclerosis and cardiovascular disease. There are three classes of lipids—triglycerides, cholesterol and cholesterol esters, and phospholipids.

Since lipids are insoluble in water it is only the weak binding ability of these agents to specific proteins that enables them to be soluble in the plasma as 'lipoproteins'. There are four classes of lipoproteins—chylomicrons, very low density lipoprotein (VLDL), low density lipoprotein (LDL), and high density lipoprotein (HDL). The chylomicrons and VLDL are rich in triglycerides while the HDL's are poor in triglycerides and the LDL's are rich in cholesterol. Atherosclerotic cardiovascular disease is associated with hypercholesterolaemia and a significant rise in LDL.

Progestogens have, to a variable extent, the capacity to reverse oestrogen-induced changes of serum lipids and lipoproteins with the possible exception of triglycerides. Norethisterone acetate has the greatest capacity to offset oestrogen effects in serum triglyceride and HDL-cholesterol. Much more research is required to sort out the relative advantages and disadvantages of various oestrogenic and progestogenic steroids in terms of atherogenicity or anti-atherogenic effects.

A large multicentre study has been carried out (Wahl et al 1983) which showed that the potency of oestrogen and progestogen in oral contraceptives must be balanced to avoid changes in LDLs and HDLs. Preparations studied in the 10 centres included equine oestrogen, ethinyloestradiol, and diethylstilboestrol in a non-menstruating group, and seven oral contraceptive formulations in a larger, menstruating group. It was found that the following results could be demonstrated:

1. HDL cholesterol levels were highest in oestrogen dominant preparations in menstruating women where the lowest HDL values were found with progestogen dominant contraceptives. In some instances these levels were below that of controls
2. LDL concentrations were highest among those using low dose oestrogen and lowest among those taking oestrogen dominant oral contraceptives

3. VLDL cholesterol levels were elevated in all oral contraceptive users

4. Triglycerides were raised by the oestrogen component of oral contraceptives and lowered by some progestogens

High LDL cholesterol has been correlated positively with the risk of coronary artery disease. In this study these authors found the highest LDL and lowest HDL values occurred in users of contraceptives containing norgestrel and norethisterone acetate. Are users of these formulations at risk from atherosclerotic cardiovascular disease?

Pseudopregnancy with combination oral contraceptives—Brisbane series

Since Sampson stated more than 50 years ago that pregnancy lessened the incidence of endometriosis and that post-pregnancy involution changes possibly retarded future development or even caused regression of implants already present, there has been much speculation about the relationship between pregnancy and endometriosis. The significant number of patients in the Brisbane series who were parous at the time of diagnosis, the evidence from Wheeler & Malinak that pregnancy does not prevent but merely delays the onset of recurrent endometriosis, and the fact that in some patients in the Brisbane series the disease actually progressed despite the effect of pregnancy and lactation, suggests a very indefinite relationship between endometriosis and the decidual changes and hyperhormonal changes of pregnancy.

The advocacy by Kistner of the use of the newer progestogens in the non-surgical treatment of endometriosis had much theoretical merit, aiming to induce decidual transformation with hyperhormonal amenorrhoea achieved by using continuous high dose oral contraceptive preparations. In the early days of the Brisbane series before laparoscopic surgery commenced, patients with stage I–II disease were offered continuous therapy with either Anovlar (ethinyloestradiol 50 µg and norethisterone acetate 4 mg), Eugyon (ethinyloestradiol 50 µg and norgestrel 500 µg) or Norinyl-I (mestranol 50 µg and norethisterone 1 mg) using two to four tablets daily in order to produce amenorrhoea.

Side-effects were unacceptably high and led to many patients dropping out of this programme and the pregnancy yield was poor (Table 6.5).

Table 6.5 Pseudopregnancy therapy—oral contraceptives used in the Brisbane series

	Total	Pregnancy	Side-effects	Persistent disease
Anovlar	31	4	26	23
Eugynon	11	1	9	9
Norinyl-I	14	3	3	7
Totals	56	8 (14%)	38 (68%)	39 (69%)

Significantly only a few of these 56 patients showed clinical improvement and the publications in the lay press of the risks of thromboembolic and cardiovascular complications associated with oestrogen-containing oral contraceptives at that time, led to the abandonment of this oral contraceptive programme in the early 1970s.

However, there is a place for modification of Kistner's ideas in routine oral contraceptive prescribing, especially in young girls with a family history of endometriosis. Reduction in the number of menses per year ought to be associated with a reduced likelihood of the development of endometriosis. Therefore, as was suggested by a postgraduate trainee in the Brisbane practice, modified oral contraceptive prescribing now consists of offering patients the choice of taking active combined contraceptive pills for 3–4 months without a break, depending on cycle control, since breakthrough bleeding may defeat the purpose of the exercise.

In 1980, Andrews recommended confining the use of pseudopregnancy to patients with early disease, not yet in a position to conceive. Kable & Yussman (1981) were of a similar opinion after reviewing 140 cases of endometriosis treated by pseudopregnancy with a post-therapy pregnancy rate of only 23%. It is in this recommended group that modified pseudopregnancy was most used in the Brisbane series.

Although Hammond et al (1976) thought there was no particular advantage in using hormonal pseudopregnancy because their best results came from conservative surgery alone, some sort of delaying tactics are needed to prevent recurrent endometriosis, if possible, after initial conservative primary surgery, especially in view of the results of conservative surgery alone in the Brisbane series.

Pseudopregnancy with progestogens alone

Since the side-effects of oral contraceptives had caused intolerable problems, mainly because of the oestrogenic fraction, it seemed reasonable in the Brisbane series to pursue the concept of progestin pseudopregnancy only. Grant (1963) had favourably reviewed the

119

effects of northisterone on endometriosis and this relatively inexpensive progestogenic agent was freely available in Brisbane at the start of the series. It became the initial continuous medication, used in doses from 5 to 20 mg daily, depending on the severity of the disease and the intended duration of the course of therapy. In most cases it has been found that, following primary conservative surgery, maintenance of progestogen-induced amenorrhoea with only 5 mg of norethisterone daily is possible for 2 to 6 months at a time, while contraceptive protection is also provided.

The basic optimal treatment for endometriosis is prolonged cessation of menstruation, preferably as the result of pregnancy. But where this cannot be achieved, continuous progestogen therapy is an acceptable alternative means to the same end of minimizing symptoms and signs (Kistner 1975), and preventing recurrence or extension of disease, thus preserving subsequent fertility.

Medroxyprogesterone acetate

The author was peripherally involved with the trials in Brisbane using an injectable form of medroxyprogesterone acetate as a contraceptive measure. Khoo et al (1971) reported on injectable medroxyprogesterone acetate and noted suppression of glandular proliferative activity in the endometrium with decidual reaction and they reported that this endometrial quiescence was reversible. Since 1970 when 1 ml ampoules of Depo-Provera 150 mg became available, this form of medroxyprogesterone acetate has been used extensively in the medical treatment of endometriosis, as well as for contraception for those patients for whom fertility is not yet, or no longer, a consideration, for those who require postsurgical medical therapy, and especially those having radical surgery where post-oophorectomy symptoms need to be blocked.

Rosenfield (1974) drew attention to long-acting progestogens as therapy for endometriosis and pointed out the safety of these preparations. He noted the mode of action was both central in the hypothalamo-pituitary axis, and peripheral in endometrial tissue, reducing glandular activity and producing thin inactive endometrium. The central action was thought to be due either to blocking the gonadotrophins, abolishing gonadotrophin surges, and blocking ovulation, since corpora lutea commonly failed to appear with this form of therapy, or, by a 'shock' effect in the hypothalamus within 24 hours of administration of the injection, and this inhibitory shock effect perhaps lasted 3 to 4 months after administration of the drug.

When reporting on a double-blind randomized placebo control study of Depo-Provera in 48 subjects, Morrison et al (1980) showed only two who received no benefit from this form of progestogen therapy in controlling menopausal symptoms. Schiff et al (1980) reported a similar trial using oral medroxyprogesterone acetate in 32 women at a daily dose of 20 mg orally. In addition to symptomatic relief, these workers found a fall in gondaotrophin levels which, on further research (Albrecht et al 1981), was found to be associated with a reduction in pulsatile LH production. Neither investigative team suggested that medroxyprogesterone acetate had a role in improving vaginal atrophy or reducing the incidence of osteoporosis but the sensible, legitimate use of this preparation is now well established, especially in patients for whom oestrogens are contra-indicated because of breast cancer, thromboembolic disease, etc.

Injectible preparations offer the advantages of freedom from daily pill taking and regular physican contact at the time of follow-up injection. The major disadvantage is the loss of ability to change one's mind about the therapy once the injection has been administered.

In the Brisbane series the results of the use of both norethisterone (and norethisterone acetate), and medroxyprogesterone acetate are similar and, in both cases, are far superior to danazol in terms of promoting fertility, controlling spread of disease, side-effects, and cost. The feared delay in the return of fertility after medroxyproges-terone acetate injections was never realized as all patients had recovery of menstruation within 12 months of receiving their last injection. This finding was in keeping with Fraser and Weisberg (1981) who noted recovery commencing about 90 days after each injection was given. Where atrophic break-through bleeding proved troublesome, a short course or two of ethinyloestradiol 0.02 mg twice daily for 25 days was usually curative.

Oral medroxyprogesterone acetate provides the opportunity to test for patient acceptability or idiosyncratic side-effects before commencing long-term Depo-Provera injection therapy. It has also been used successfully (Moghissi & Boyce 1976) in the treatment of endometriosis previously and in the Brisbane series was often used where short-term therapy only was required. No sinister long-term side-effects have been noticed in the Brisbane series, some patients having been on continuous Depo-Provera injection therapy now for up to 10 years, enjoying a 'menses free' and 'endometriosis free' existence without side-effects. Toppozada et al (1978) reported that norethisterone oenanthate has, like Depo-Provera, no effect on

LHRH response and they believe the suppressive action of both preparations is at a level of the hypothalamus or higher and, although the clinical responses of both vary differently in time scale of events, both coincide in contraceptive effectiveness and presumably in anti-endometriosis effect. Unfortunately, injectible norethisterone oenanthate is not available in Brisbane.

Norethisterone and norethisterone acetate

When these drugs were used in the continuous progestin programme for the treatment of endometriosis in the Brisbane series, some patients dropped out because of side-effects of depression, weight gain, sebaceous skin problems, or loss of a feeling of well-being. The acetate from was used for more extensive disease because of its enhanced progestogenic activity. In the Brisbane series the ready availability and inexpensive cost factor of these drugs led to their extensive use in the early years and whether these drugs or medroxyprogesterone acetate are used now, depends on a fairly arbitrary assessment of anticipated patient response, based in part on prior reaction to oral contraceptives of known chemical constitution, and response to trial doses of these progestins.

It has been claimed that there is a significant endogenous conversion of norethisterone to oestrogenic substances. This theory has not been borne out by the Brisbane series but has resulted in some endometriosis patients in the past, being denied access to this very useful drug programme. As can be seen by the results of treatment in the Brisbane series, these are very effective aids to surgery in the management of endometriosis.

Dydrogesterone

Dydrogesterone has been used extensively in the treatment of endometriosis by Johnston (1976) and his co-workers in Melbourne. It is also mentioned without expansion by Venter (1980) as an agent that can be used to treat endometriosis. As Duphaston 10 mg tablets it has recently been made available in Australia with a Commonwealth Government subsidy for the treatment of surgically proven endometriosis. Although dydrogesterone is said to be relatively free of anabolic, androgenic, or oestrogenic side-effects, Johnston, while claiming excellent results in terms of symptom relief and improved culdoscopic appearance post-treatment, did note three patients in whom the disease progressed despite therapy, with the development of new deposits. Since it has been stated that dydrogesterone does not produce endometrial atrophy or dedidual reaction, the mode of action in its anti-endometriosis role remains obscure, and is the reason why it has not been pursued in the Brisbane series, although it remains an option to take up when other, better tested, progestogens can no longer be continued because of side-effects.

Pseudomenopause therapy

Danocrine (Danazol/Danol)

Danazol was first described as an antigonadotrophin derived from ethisterone by Greenblatt et al (1971) and since that time there has been a flood of literature concerning Danazol; several international symposia have discussed it, and practitioners and patients have hoped—in vain—that it would prove to be the much needed medical panacea for endometriosis.

While the alleged antigonadotrophic activity would seem to have mainly been just a blockage of mid-cycle LH surge, more recent studies by Bevan et al (1984) suggest that danazol is not an antigonadotrophin in terms of resulting biological effects, but rather works by lowering sex hromone binding globulin levels.

Mildwisky et al (1983) demonstrated evidence, based on competition analysis, that danazol had the ability to displace androgen from androgen high affinity binders, and progesterone from progesterone high affinity binders in cytosol from residual ovarian syndrome oophorectomy specimens. This they suggested was evidence of a possible direct action of danazol on the human ovary.

Having previously authored and co-authored many papers dealing with danazol, Dmowski (1981), in a then current review of this drug in relation to endometriosis, mentioned the variability of results of laboratory studies with regard to danazol and gonadotrophin production, although the clinical effect produced by danazol was markedly antigonadotrophic. Plasma oestriol levels were noted to be almost undetectable, plasma progesterone levels were low, and endometrium showed epithelial thinning and glandular and stromal atrophy. Similar histological changes were demonstrated in endometriotic tissue (Greenblatt et al 1971) and small thin walled endometrioma showed a clinical response, while larger thick walled lesions were relatively insensitive to danazol. Jenkin (1980) also believed that a factor other than antigonadotrophic properties accounted for the efficacy of danazol in other conditions as well as

123

endometriosis, while Barbieri & Ryan (1981) believed that because of the complex pharmacology exhibited by danazol, it was inappropriate to continue to refer to it as 'a selective antigonadotrophin'.

The results from using danazol in the Brisbane series were seriously disappointing. Not only was there little clinical or surgical improvement in endometriosis, but infertility was not markedly improved. Only four of 20 patients who wished to conceive did so within 6–12 months of ceasing therapy with this drug. On the other hand, 55 of 65 patients using danazol experienced side-effects sufficiently severe in 60% of cases for them not to complete more than 3 months of therapy. As a consequence of this experience, danazol is no longer used as a first drug of choice in the conservative management of endometriosis.

This was at total variance with the experience of Dmowski & Cohen (1975) who using laparoscopy before and after reported very impressive findings where only 15% of their 39 patients showed clinical or histological endometriosis following danazol therapy only, with no previous surgery other than laparoscopy/biopsy. In their series, 59% had no evidence of disease and 26% had peritoneal adhesions and haemosiderin deposits but no active disease. Cohen (1980) and Jenkin (1980) mention the high cost factor when danazol is prescribed in both the USA and Australia and danazol, which costs the Australian tax payer more than $A1 per 200 mg tablet, only became available in Australia for the treatment of endometriosis with a Commonwealth Government subsidy in 1978, provided the disease had been operatively proven. One hopes that in future, reports in the international literature of results of treatment of endometriosis will only include those cases operatively proven.

Anxieties that long-term danazol usage was associated with atherogenic changes in cholesterol and HDL lipoproteins were first voiced by Fraser & Allen in 1979 following their study of a group of patients taking various danazol dosages for over 6 months. Cohen (1980) shared these anxieties and Allen & Fraser (1981) confirmed their initial report that danazol suppresses HDL-cholesterol levels and elevates the levels of cholesterol and other lipid protein fractions. Further confirmatory work was published in 1983 by Luciano et al who showed, in a study of patients on danazol at doses as low as 200 mg daily, that within 4 weeks of starting therapy, there was a fall in HDL with recovery taking up to 4 weeks after cessation of therapy. This would suggest that especially in the genetically vulnerable, and in obese, physically indolent, cigarette smokers the risk of atherogenic cardiovascular disease must increase if danazol is prescribed.

In therapeutic doses, danazol has a half-life of 4.5 h (Williams et al 1978) so therapy has always been given in divided doses to try and achieve the best effects. Cohen (1980) and Dmowski (1981) believed danazol serves its best primary therapeutic role in mild to moderate disease where patients are infertile. Cohen also mentions those patients who cannot tolerate other medications—the only situation in which the drug is now used in the Brisbane series.

In terms of fertility outcome the news is not all good. Siebel et al (1982) in a controlled study showed that there was a 30% conception rate in a danazol treated infertile group and a 50% conception rate in a group treated by conservative surgery alone. They suggested that danazol had a limited place in the early postoperative phase of treatment after surgery for endometriosis associated with infertility.

Greenblatt and Tzingounis (1979) studied a group of 30 patients wanting pregnancy, and 10 of 20 patients with potential fertility conceived after danazol therapy.

Puleo and Hammond (1983) reported a 50% conception rate in their series while Wheeler and Malinak (1981), in a large series of 200 women with severe endometriosis divided into two study groups—conservative surgery alone and conservative surgery followed by danazol—found the conception rate for surgery alone to be 36 out of 119 (30%) and 15 out of 19 (79%) for those having danazol. However, only 21% of this second smaller group had coexistent infertility factors such as fibroids, anovulation, cervical factors, male factors etc, compared with 47% of the group not receiving danazol and having the lower conception rate.

Daniell and Christianson (1981) treated 66 patients with a combination of laparoscopy and danazol and reported a corrected fertility rate of 68%. They noted that the majority of pregnancy successes occurred within six months of therapy. Moore et al (1981) used a low dose danazol programme and reported a successful conception rate of 28%.

In a comparative study using danazol in 27, and Enovid in 23 patients with proved endometriosis, Noble & Letchworth (1980) found that nine of 16 wishing to become pregnant in the danazol group succeeded (56% success rate) and four of 11 of the Enovid group conceived (36% success rate). They believed danazol produced dramatic clinical improvement in endometriosis patients who did not have advanced disease but they did report one danazol user with voice changes complicating therapy.

Recurrence after treatment has been reported as between 25 and 39% (Dmowski 1979, Ward 1979, Greenblatt and Tzingounis 1979, Biberoglu & Behrman 1981, Puleo & Hammond 1983). In fact Dmowski reported an average annual recurrence rate of 39% compared with that of 15% in patients treated by either surgery or pseudopregnancy. Biberoglu & Behrman believed that the 36% symptomatic recurrence rate they reported was dose dependent as they had treated some patients with daily doses as low as 100 mg per day to study long-term effectiveness on amelioration of surgically confirmed endometriosis. The low-dose programme of Moore et al (1981) was associated with a recurrence rate of 54% within 1 year of cessation of danazol.

Mettler & Semm (1979) and van Zyl et al (1980) have reported favourably on a triphasic therapeutic programme of surgery, danazol and review surgery. The latter group found a complete cure in 42% of patients treated with danazol but when the timing of danazol was altered to immediately after conservative surgery the number completely cured at review rose to 60%.

Throughout the many reports of danazol therapy there is mention of side-effects which are usually qualified with adjectives such as 'mild', 'minimal', 'well tolerated', 'trivial'. Dmowski in his review (1981) states that danazol-induced pseudomenopause therapy produced 'few, rather well tolerated, side-effects'. This was not the experience in Brisbane and, in fact, 60% of patients in the Brisbane series did not continue beyond 3 months of therapy because of side-effects which were experienced by 55 of 65 danazol users (85%) and were regarded by most, as severe (not mild) and major (not minor).

The production of a sudden chemical menopause-like state in a previously robust young female has serious emotional, as well as, physical side-effects. One articulate, intelligent medical graduate patient described the feeling while on danazol as being 'neutered'. Most patients found that hot flushes from vasomotor instability and pruritus vulvae associated with atrophic genital epithelium changes in the subtropical climate of Brisbane were totally unacceptable. A high incidence of vocal cord hypertrophy and voice change (12%) was critically important and an embarrassing side-effect to those who experienced it, especially in teachers, singers etc. whose daily work depended on voice function and communication with the public. One patient still has this problem 2 years after the cessation of danazol.

All side-effects were far worse in those patients having coexistent polycystic ovary disease and in them the exaggerated androgenic properties (dramatically compounded weight gain, skin problems, anabolic effects and personality problems) were very slow to resolve.

If after these unacceptable side-effects in danazol users the result had been a high success rate in terms of cure or successful pregnancy in those who were infertile, some justification for use could be offered. In fact only four of the 20 danazol users wishing to do so and who had no other infertility factors, had conceived within 6 months of completing danazol therapy. A comparison of the side-effects between the drugs commonly used in the Brisbane series is shown in Table 6.6.

It seems amazing that Barbieri et al (1982) in their series of 100 patients treated with danazol, of whom 85 experienced side-effects, had only one who dropped out. In the Brisbane series 36 of 65 danazol users dropped out because of side-effects. In terms of cure, only three of the 65 patients who used danazol have remained clinically free of disease and required no further therapy. Eleven have been lost to follow-up, undoubtedly because of the experience of side-effects. A further 43 patients have required further surgery and treatment with other medical modalities. The economic waste to the community runs into thousands of dollars and the disappointment and side-effects suffered by users of this drug, prescribed with the best of intentions, is horrific beyond acceptable bounds.

An excellent comparative study of the effects of pseudomenopause using danazol and of medical oophorectomy using a gonadotrophin releasing hormone (GnRH) agonist in two small groups, each of five patients with proven endometriosis, was published by Meldrum et al (1983). Danazol consumption was at the recommended oral dosage of 400 mg 12-hourly and GnRH agonist was given in a dose of 100 µg subcutaneously, daily at 0800 h for 28 days beginning on day 5 of the menstrual cycle. A further five previously oophorectomized women also had blood samples taken for comparisons. In all three groups serum oestrone, oestradiol, and testosterone levels were recorded along with levels of sex hormone binding globulins.

Danazol treatment was associated with a reduction of the mean level of oestradiol compared to pretreatment and throughout the 6 months of danazol therapy, limited maturation of ovarian follicles was reflected in infrequent serum oestradiol elevations. With the maximum recommended daily dose of danazol the mean oestradiol concentration was equivalent to the lower range seen in premenopausal women in the follicular phase of menstrual cycles, and was three times greater than the levels in oophorectomized women.

Daily injections of GnRH analogue reduced total oestrone and

Table 6.6 Side-effects of medical treatment of endometriosis in the Brisbane series

	Danazol	Norethisterone	Norethisterone acetate	Depo-Provera	Provera	Oral contraceptives	Totals
Depression	32	18	6	36	7	17	116
Weight gain	28	11	6	38	10	16	109
Acne	22	6	4	20	7	13	72
Vaginal bleeding	5	23	3	15	5	20	71
Headaches	10	4	1	12	4	4	35
Libido	18	4	3	5	1	1	32
Defeminization	24	0	1	0	0	1	26
Breast changes	5	4	2	6	0	8	25
Pruritus vulvae	19	0	1	1	0	3	24
Voice changes	9	1	0	0	0	0	10
Hot flushes	5	0	0	0	0	0	8
Other	4†	0	2*	7‡	3	6	22
Total side-effects	181	71	32	140	37	89	550
Total patients with side-effects	55	44	11	23	15	38	186
Total drug users	65	122	19	171	35	87	499

† 2: clitoral hypertrophy; * 1 patient with galactorrhoea; ‡ 2 patients with galactorrhoea
Depo-Provera: medroxyprogesterone acetate 150 mg/ml depot injection
Provera: medroxyprogesterone acetate 10 mg tablets

oestradiol concentrations to levels that were one-third to one-half those recorded during danazol therapy, and similar to those of oophorectomized women. The mechanism of this effect is complex and in part due to the GnRH analogue markedly suppressing follicle stimulating hormone production. In this regard it appears that danazol suppresses ovarian steroidogenesis while GnRH eliminates ovarian oestrogen secretion, thus effecting a medically induced oophrectomy state.

In this study, danazol therapy was also associated with marked reduction in sex hormone binding globulin to almost undetectable levels. This reduction would then be expected to increase the tissue availability of both oestradiol and testosterone. The level of free oestradiol at the end of danazol therapy was up to five times that of oophorectomized women while, on the other hand, GnRH agonist treatment had no effect on sex hormone binding globulin concentration and reduced the free oestradiol level to lower than that with danazol therapy, and similar to that of oophorectomized women.

The generalization reached about danazol therapy by these workers was that it produced uniform low levels of oestradiol, almost undetectable levels of sex hormone binding globulin, and a marked increase in free testosterones. GnRH analogue therapy suppressed ovarian function and reduced oestrone and free oestradiol to levels only one-quarter to one-half those of oophorectomized females. These results suggested that suppression of ovarian function using GnRH analogue may have an effect on endometriosis similar to bilateral oophrectomy while avoiding the androgenic side-effects of danazol.

Medical oophrectomy
(based on a contribution by Professor Robert Shaw)

Professor R W Shaw of the Royal Free Hospital, London, has kindly responded to the Publisher's request for assistance and has supplied valuable information concerning the use of luteinizing hormone releasing hormone agonists as a possible new approach in endometriosis therapy including the results of treatment in a series of 18 patients under his care.

Surgical castration, as mentioned previously, has traditionally been the most effective form of treatment of endometriosis. Recently, gonadal function suppression in a reversible fashion has been demonstrated following daily administration of long-acting luteinizing hormone releasing hormone (LHRH) agonists ($LHRH_A$)

129

(Bergquist et al 1979). It has been suggested that the ability of LHRH$_A$ to produce a reversible medical oophorectomy by ovarian suppression may emerge as a new approach in the medical management of endometriosis, conferring the advantages of bilateral surgical oophorectomy with the conservation of ovarian tissue and potential fertility.

Effect of LHRH agonists on gonadotrophin secretion

LHRH is a polypeptide containing 10 amino acid residues. Naturally occurring LHRH is degraded in the hypothalamus (Hersh & McKelvy 1979) and pituitary gland (Koch et al 1974), by peptidases which cleave molecules at the Gly^6–Leu^7 bond and at position 9.

A large number of LHRH$_A$ has been synthesized with a D-amino acid substituted into position 6 and often with an ethylamide group in place of the terminal glycinamide residue (Coy et al 1976). These analogues have a reduced susceptibility to enzymatic degradation and therefore have prolonged biological—and potentially therapeutic—activity, in addition to high binding affinity to LHRH receptors.

Recent publications include long-term studies of prolonged LHRH$_A$ treatment in humans and primates showing that those pituitary cells secreting FSH and LH become insensitive to continuing stimulation with such agents leading to a suppression of ovarian steroid secretion (Schmidt-Gollwitzer et al 1981, Bergquist et al 1982, Fraser 1982).

In postmenopausal women continuing LHRH$_A$ administration results in marked suppression of circulating FSH and LH and blunted pituitary responsiveness to endogenous LHRH administration (Shaw et al 1985 Fig. 6.4).

In premenopausal females, following a transient period of increased gonadotrophin secretion lasting some days, further increase in gonadotrophins in response to LHRH$_A$ administration is abolished. Although circulating levels of FSH return to basal levels quickly, serum LH tends to be maintained above basal levels (Lemay et al 1984). There is, however, a loss of pulsatile gonadotrophin secretion (R W Shaw unpublished data) and it may well be this disruption of pulsatile gonadotrophin signal which is responsible for the suppression of ovarian oestrogen secretion and not an absolute need to reduce significantly circulating FSH and LH levels.

In 1982 Meldrum et al published the results of treating five patients with endometriosis with daily subcutaneous injection of

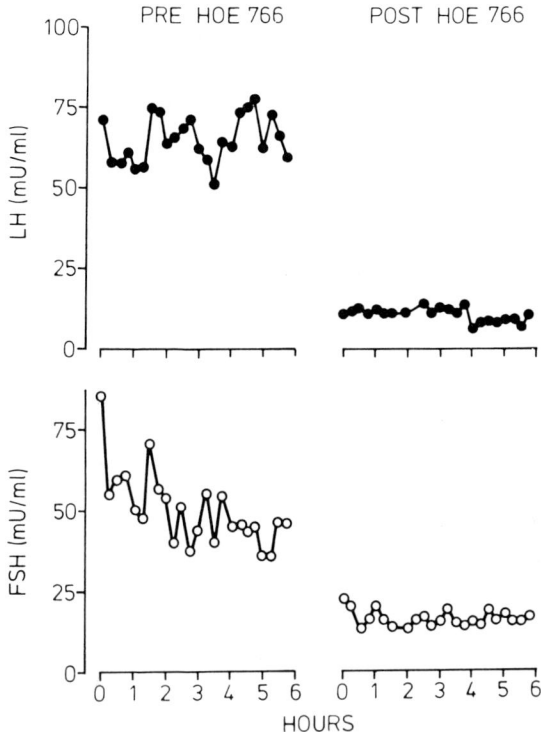

Fig. 6.4 Suppression of basal levels and abolition of pulsatile pattern of release of LH and FSH in a postmenopausal female receiving the LHRH agonist (HOE 766) Buserelin, 200 µg twice daily intranasally for 21 days. (Reproduced by kind permission Professor R W Shaw and Maturitas 7:161–167 1985)

100 µg of $LHRH_A$-D-Trp^6-Pro^9-Net LHRH for 28 days using five oophorectomized women as controls.

They found that the treated women showed an increased oestradiol secretion for some 2 weeks after which serum oestradiol fell below castrate values in the third and fourth weeks. Each patient had vaginal bleeding within 1 week of the fall in oestrogen level and at the end of treatment as well as in the following cycle. All five patients reported complete disappearance of, or improvement in, premenstrual pain, dyspareunia and dyschezia. Periods returned 25–31 days after the completion of therapy with biphasic basal temperature chart patterns in the cycle after therapy. This study was really a 'sighting shot' in the endometriosis battle but seemed to be pointed at a new method of achieving the desired post-oophorectomy castration state without surgery.

131

Also in 1982 Lemay and Quesnel used the LHRH agonist D-Ser (TBU)^6-des Gly-NH$_2$^{10}LHRH ethylamide (Buserelin) 300 μg twice daily in an endometriosis sufferer for 6 months and noted that suppression of ovarian steroid secretion was associated not only with improvement in the severity of the endometriosis symptoms but also in a reduction of the number of endometriosis deposits.

Further definitive studies using Buserelin intranasally in doses of 200 μg three times a day (Shaw et al 1983), 200 μg twice daily subcutaneously for 5 days and then intranasally 400 μg three times daily (Lemay et al 1984) and a comparison between 200 μg three times a day and 300 μg three times a day intranasally (Shaw & Fraser 1984) have confirmed the initial hopes of a therapeutic value for LHRH$_A$ in the treatment of endometriosis. The work done by Professor Shaw and his colleagues involved patients whose endometriosis had been confirmed at laparoscopy and staged according to the American Fertility Society classification (see ch. 4). Their patients commenced Buserelin at a dose of 200 μg three times a day (eight patients) and 300 μg three times a day (10 patients) intranasally between days 1 to 3 of their cycle and treatment was continued for 6 months. After this time repeat laparoscopy was used to re-evaluate the disease staging and response to treatment.

Circulating oestradiol levels

At both dose levels of Buserelin the mean circulating serum oestradiol was significantly reduced ($P < 0.001$) after 4 weeks of treatment from that in the pretreatment (mid-luteal) phase. Continuing suppression of serum oestradiol was achieved throughout therapy although some patients receiving the lower dose showed bursts of follicular activity with rises in oestrogen levels (Fig. 6.5).

This type of response was not seen with the higher dose regimen.

When serum oestradiol values were maintained at levels consistently within the menopausal range (less than 90 pmol/l) then hot flushes and sweats developed in most individuals and the frequency, intensity, and duration seemed to be dose related (Table 6.7).

Other menopausal-type symptoms related to oestrogen deficiency—dry vagina, superficial dyspareunia, breast atrophy and loss of libido—were also found to develop, but only in individuals with extreme oestradiol suppression—values of less than 50 pmol/l. The fact that not every individual, even with these low oestradiol values, developed symptoms was probably related to the relatively short duration of ovarian suppression.

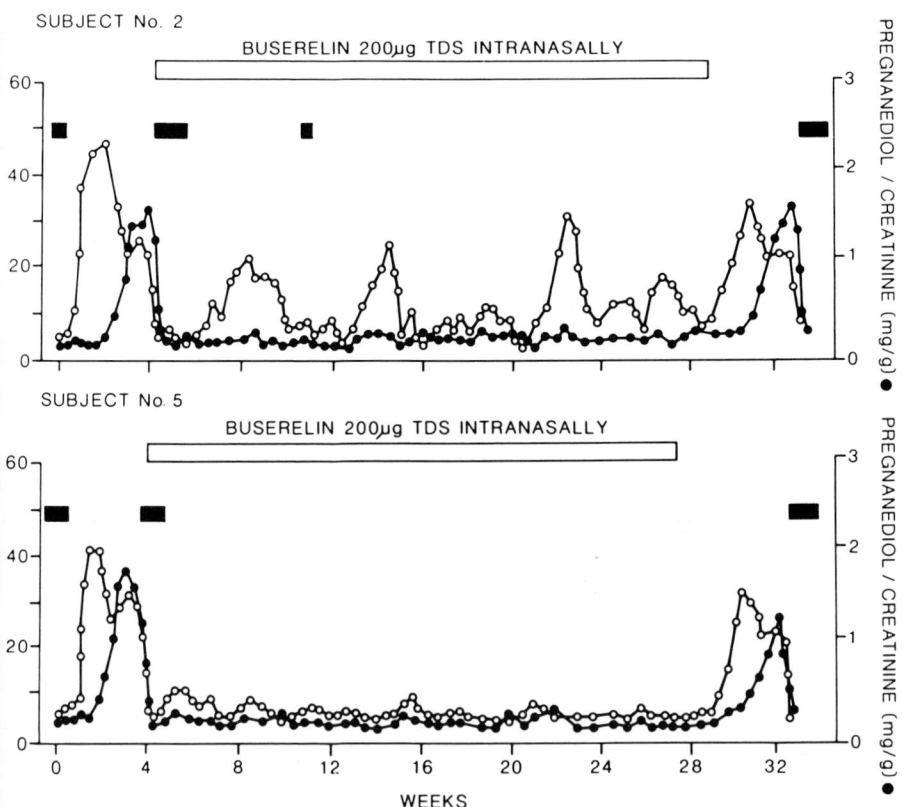

Fig. 6.5 Patterns of urinary steroid excretion in two patients receiving Buserelin 200 μg three times daily intranasally for 6 months. ■ ■ = episodes of menstrual bleeding. (Reproduced by kind permission Professor R W Shaw and British Medical Journal 1983 287 : 1667–1669)

Uterine bleeding patterns

During the first 6 weeks of therapy 11 of the 18 patients in Professor Shaw's series reported some episodes of menstrual bleeding between days 18 and 38 on treatment which corresponded to oestrogen withdrawal. Only four of the 18 reported any further bleeding episodes during the remainder of treatment and all episodes were minimal. These findings were not dissimilar to those of Meldrum et al (1982) in their smaller series.

Endometrial biopsies at the end of 6 months of therapy were consistently reported as 'atrophic endometrium' although three of

Table 6.7 Circulating serum oestradiol levels during LHRH agonist treatment with D-Ser (TBu)⁶-des Gly-NH₂¹⁰LHRH ethylamide (Buserelin) and the incidence of patients experiencing hot flushes (Reproduced by kind permission Professor R W Shaw)

Month of treatment	Buserelin 200 μg t.d.s. intranasally (n = 8)		Buserelin 300 μg t.d.s. intranasally (n = 10)	
	Serum oestradiol (pmol/l: mean ± s.e.m.)	No. of patients with hot flushes	Serum oestradiol (pmol/l: mean ± s.e.m.)	No. of patients with hot flushes
Pretreatment	382 ± 64	—	401 ± 32	—
2	124 ± 19	0/8	84 ± 17	4/10
4	105 ± 37	1/8	62 ± 21	6/9
6	110 ± 28	2/8	64 ± 16	8/9
Post-treatment	296 ± 86	—	284 ± 68	—

t.d.s. : three times daily

the patients on Professor Shaw's programme of 200 μg three times a day had poorly developed proliferative phase endometrium. Four cases yielded no endometrium whatsoever at curettage.

The patients in Meldrum's series had return of menstruation 25–31 days after completion of therapy, while those in Professor Shaw's series similarly had first menstruation at a mean of 32 ± 6.4 days after cessation of $LHRH_A$.

Circulating progesterone concentrations suggested that it is invariably an ovulatory cycle on recovery, indicating a readily reversible form of ovarian inhibition (see Fig. 6.6).

Symptoms of endometriosis

Eleven of the 18 patients in the Shaw et al series had mild to moderate dysmenorrhoea prior to treatment and at 6 months post-treatment follow-up, the severity was unchanged in one, improved in five, and had disappeared in five. All had complete relief on treatment even if menstruation had occurred.

Deep dyspareunia, a significant complaint in six of the 18 patients was relieved by the end of 3 months' treatment in five patients (83%) but persisted in the remaining patient. Superficial dyspareunia due to reduced circulating oestradiol levels was a complication during treatment in three patients, a problem similar to that found with danazol treatment in patients in other series.

Pain—premenstrual and intermenstrual—present before treatment was found by Professor Shaw to be alleviated in all seven sufferers after 4 months of LHRH$_A$ treatment. Five of the seven remained free of pain 6 months after the cessation of therapy while further LHRH$_A$ treatment was effective in controlling post-treatment pain episodes in the others.

Changes in endometriotic deposits

Twelve of 18 patients in Professor Shaw's series had abnormal gynaecological findings on pelvic examination with tenderness and/ or nodules in the pouch of Douglas. Post treatment, all but one patient with persistent palpable utero-sacral ligament nodules were normal on gynaecological review examination.

Table 6.8 demonstrates the laparoscopic findings and staging before and after treatment of 17 of the 18 patients in Professor Shaw's series. Small endometriotic implants invariably underwent complete resolution while large deposits demonstrated a reduction in size. Staging took into account adhesion formation in addition to endometriotic lesions and in cases where adhesions contributed materially to the staging, improvement was far less apparent. This finding would suggest that LHRH$_A$ will find its most useful role in the treatment of stage 0 and I lesions where adhesion formation is minimal.

Table 6.8 Laparoscopic findings, staging and scoring of endometriosis before and following 6 months' therapy with D-Ser (TBu)[6]-des Gly NH$_2$[10]-LHRH ethylamide (Buserelin) (Reproduced by kind permission Professor R W Shaw)

Buserelin 200 µg t.d.s. intranasally				Buserelin 300 µg t.d.s. intranasally			
Patient no.	American Fertility Society classification (stage)		Endometriosis implants only (total points)	Patient no.	American Fertility Society classification (stage)		Endometriosis implants only (total points)
	Before	After	Before	After		Before	After	Before	After
1	I	0	5	0	1	I	With-drawn	4	With-drawn
2	II	0	4	0	2	I	0	2	0
3	II	0	5	0	3	II	0	4	0
4	III	II	6	2	4	III	II	6	1
5	IV	III	7	1	5	II	0	4	0
6	I	0	2	0	6	IV	III	6	1
7	I	0	4	0	7	I	0	2	0
8	II	0	5	0	8	II	0	6	0
					9	II	I	8	2
					10	II	0	4	0

t.d.s.: three times daily

Conclusions

These reported studies to date demonstrate that treatment with LHRH$_A$ is useful in suppressing ovarian steroid hormone production and by utilizing appropriate dose programmes, the circulating oestrogen levels can be reduced to menopausal levels thereby producing a reversible 'medical oophorectomy' (Table 6.9).

Table 6.9 The effects of various medical treatment approaches on endometrial tissue (Reproduced by kind permission Professor R W Shaw)

	Effect on endometrium	Effect on endometrial deposits
Oestrogen	Proliferation Hyperplasia	Proliferation Hyperplasia
Progesterone	Growth arrest Secretory changes Decidual reaction	Growth arrest Secretory changes Decidual reaction Necrobiosis
Androgens	Atrophy	Atrophy and regression
Oophorectomy (lack of oestrogen)	Atrophy	Atrophy and regression
LHRH agonists	Poor proliferative growth or atrophy	Atrophy and regression

Signs and symptoms of oestrogen deficiency were the only side-effects noted in these reported series and in some instances they were of significant inconvenience to the patients, perhaps similar to side-effects experienced with hormonal therapies, but possibly less troublesome.

The resorption of endometriosis deposits correlated, according to Professor Shaw's series, with a marked inhibition of ovarian follicular activity, and associated symptoms related to the disease were also significantly relieved. With currently available treatment some patients have recurrence of endometriosis once therapy is stopped. Long-term follow-up studies after the use of LHRH agonists are not yet available to ascertain whether these offer significant advantages in this respect.

In addition to this new therapeutic approach to endometriosis with LHRH$_A$, Bergquist et al 1982 have used long-term intranasal LHRH$_A$ successfully for contraceptive purposes and Lemay et al (1983) suggested intranasal LHRH$_A$ at any stage between day 1–10 after the mid-cycle LH surge could lead to a new post-coital contraceptive technique acting through impairment of luteal function.

While these early experimental results with LHRH$_A$ are certainly encouraging, there is still at this time no 100% effective medical agent available for treating all cases and all stages of endometriosis.

Other agents not available in Brisbane
Gestrinone

Coutinho (1982) reported from Brazil on the usefulness of a synthetic tri-enic 19-norsteroid agent with antigonadotrophic properties that can be administered either as an intradermal implant which remains effective for one year or in a weekly 5 mg dosage. The main effects demonstrated with this drug were:

1. An affinity for progesterone receptors
2. Binding to androgen and aldosterone receptors but without a very marked antagonistic effect
3. A poorly understood anti-oestrogenic effect which counters the uterotopic effect of oestrogen without binding to oestrogen receptors.

Side-effects encountered in the 66 patients in this report included hoarse voice, breast hypotrophy, acne and sebaceous skin changes, endometrial atrophy and amenorrhoea, transient leg pain and oedema. Coutinho felt that the symptom relief and pregnancy rate compared with Danazol in the long-term, with the advantage that a twice weekly dose of 5 mg was sufficient to treat endometriosis and a once weekly dose of 5 mg was sufficient for contraception.

No matter what the stated advantages of Gestrinone, it sounds suspiciously like Danazol in terms of side-effects and even if it were available in Brisbane it would probably not attract much interest because of this.

Gossypol

Gossypol is obtained as a yellow phenolic compound from the seed, stem and root of the cotton plant and is used as 'gossypol acetate' in China. Chinese scientists had noted, by mass investigation in the 1950s, that cooking with crude cotton seed oil could lead to male infertility.

Cheng Kuo-Fen et al (1980) from Peking reported that gossypol acetate administered to women diagnosed clinically as having menorrhagia, endometriosis or fibroids, in doses of 20 mg daily for two months and 25 mg twice weekly for maintenance, produced reversible endometrial atrophy in about 50% of cases after three months of therapy. The results improved with prolongation of therapy but so did the recovery time of menses after cessation of therapy.

Another of the Peking workers reported results of treatment in 400 women to the Tenth Annual Meeting of the American Association of Gynaecological Laparoscopists in Phoenix, Arizona in November 1981. About 81 of these patients were women with endometriosis of whom two were unaffected by gossypol acetate dosage of 40 mg daily for 20 days followed by twice weekly doses for maintenance for up to six months. The others showed improvement in dysmenorrhoea (80%) and reduction of pouch of Douglas nodules (50%).

Gossypol acetate was found to be an effective reversible suppressor of FSH-LH, and recovery to normal FSH-LH levels took three months after cessation of therapy. It was thought that Gossypol also reduced the number of oestrogen and progesterone receptors in endometrium and also the endometrial content of progesterone, although it did not produce a significant fall in serum levels.

Unfortunately side-effects were sometimes serious—especially electrolyte disturbances, hypokalaemia, and altered renal and liver function.

Gossypol has also been reported by Ratsula et al (1983) to be an effective contraceptive agent when used vaginally in a gel. Studies showed dramatic sperm immobilization in 11 of 15 subjects and non-progressive reduced sperm motility in the other four. Because these workers have also been able to show that gossypol has an inhibitory effect on herpes simplex type 11 virus in vitro, they suggest that this is yet another attractive property of gossypol acetate.

Promegestone

Promegestone is a potent progestin devoid of androgenic side-effects and had marked anti-oestrogenic activity. Raynaud and Ojassoo (1983) reported on its historical research value as 'R 5020'—used extensively as a radioligand for the progestin receptor and on its therapeutic value in luteal insufficiency where in a double blind trial it was shown to be of superior potency to dydrogesterone.

On this basis it may have a future role in the therapy of endometriosis as a long-term progestogen.

REFERENCES

Albrecht B H, Schiff I, Tulchinsky D, Ryan K J 1981 Objective evidence that placebo and oral medroxyprogesterone acetate therapy diminishes menopausal vasomotor flushes. American Journal of Obstetrics and Gynecology 139:631–635

Allen J K, Fraser I 1981 Cholesterol, high density lipoprotein and danazol. Journal of Clinical Endocrinology and Metabolism 53:149–152

Andrews W C 1980 Medical versus surgical treatment of endometriosis. Clinical Obstetrics and Gynecology 23:917–924

Baggish M 1983 Status of the CO_2 laser for infertility surgery. Fertility and Sterility 40:442–445

Barbieri R C, Ryan K J 1981 Danazol: endocrine pharmacology and therapeutic applications. American Journal of Obstetrics and Gynecology 141:453–463

Barbieri R C, Evans S, Kistner R W 1982 Danazol in the treatment of endometriosis: analysis of 100 cases with a four year follow up. Fertility and Sterility 37:737–746

Beecham C T 1958 Credit for earlier statements on endometriosis and pseudo pregnancy. American Journal of Obstetrics and Gynecology 76:228 (editorial correspondence)

Bergquist C, Nillius S J, Wide L 1979 Inhibition of ovulation in women by intranasal treatment with a luteinizing hormone-releasing hormone agonist. Contraception 19:497–506

Bergquist C, Nillius S J, Wide L 1982a Intranasal LHRH agonist treatment for inhibition of ovulation in women: clinical aspects. Clinical Endocrinology 17:91–98

Bergquist C, Nillius S J, Wide C 1982b Long term intranasal LHRH agonist treatment for contraception in women. Fertility and Sterility 38:190–193

Bevan J R, Dowsett M, Jeffcoate S C 1984 Endocrine effects of danazol in the treatment of endometriosis. British Journal of Obstetrics and Gynaecology 91:160–166

Biberoglu K O, Behrman S J 1981 Dosage aspects of danazol therapy in endometriosis: short term and long term effectiveness. American Journal of Obstetrics and Gynecology 139:645–654

Brenner P 1982 The pharmacology of progestogens. Journal of Reproductive Medicine 27:409–497

Bronson R A 1977 Tubal pregnancy and infertility. Fertility and Sterility 28:221–228

Buttram V C Jr 1979a Conservative surgery for endometriosis in the infertile female. Fertility and Sterility 31:117–123

Buttram V C Jr 1979b Surgical treatment of the infertile female, a modified approach. Fertility and Sterility 32:635–640

Cheng Kuo-Fen W U, Wei Yu, Tang Min-Yi, Chu Peng-Ti 1980 Endometrial changes after the administration of gossypol for menorrhagia. American Journal of Obstetrics and Gynecology 138:1227–1229

Chong A P, Baggish M S 1984 Management of pelvic endometriosis by means of intra-abdominal carbon dioxide laser. Fertility and Sterility 41:14–19

Clark J H, Hsueh A J M, Peck E J 1977 Regulation of oestrogen receptor replenishment by progesterone. Annals of the New York Academy of Science 286:161–176

Cohen M R 1980 Laparoscopic diagnosis and pseudo menopause treatment of endometriosis with danazol. Clinical Obstetrics and Gynecology 23:901–915

Cohen M R 1982 Laparoscopy in the diagnosis and management of endometriosis. Journal of Reproductive Medicine 27:240–242

Collins J A, Wrixon W, James L B, Wilson E H 1983 Treatment—independent pregnancy among infertile couples. New England Journal of Medicine 309:1201–1206

Endometriosis

Corson S C 1979 Use of the laparoscope in the infertile patient. Fertility and Sterility 32:359–369

Counsellor V W 1949 Surgical procedures involved in the treatment of endometriosis. Surgery, Gynecology and Obstetrics 89:322–327

Coutinho E M 1982 Treatment of endometriosis with gestrinone R 2323 a synthetic anti-oestrogen, anti-progesterone. American Journal of Obstetrics and Gynecology 144:895–898

Coy D H, Vilchez-Martinez J A, Coy E J, Schally A V 1976 Analogs of luteinizing hormone-releasing hormone with increased biological activity produced by D-amino acid substitutions in position 6, Journal of Medical Chemistry 19:423–425

Craft I 1984 In vitro fertilization, clinical methodology. British Journal of Hospital Medicine 31:90–102

Cunanen R, Courey N G, Lippes J 1983 Laparoscopic findings in patients with pelvic pain. American Journal of Obstetrics and Gynecology 146:589–591

Daniell J F, Christianson C 1981 Combined laparoscopic surgery and danazol therapy for pelvic endometriosis. Fertility and Sterility 35:521–525

Diamond M, Daniell J F, McLaughlin D S, Martin D, Vaughn W K, Feste J 1984 Laser versus conventional microscopy for tubo peritoneal infertility: initial report of the intra-abdominal laser study group. Fertility and Sterility 41:465 (abstract)

Dmowski W 1979 Endocrine properties and clinical application of danazol. Fertility and Sterility 31:237–251

Dmowski W 1981 Current concepts in the management of endometriosis. Obstetrics and Gynecology Annual 279–311

Dmowski W, Cohen M R 1975 Treatment of endometriosis with an anti gondaotrophin danazol; a laparoscopic and histologic evaluation. Obstetrics and Gynecology 46:147–154

Edgren R A 1980 Progestogens. In: Givens J R (ed) Clinical use of sex steroids, Year Book Medical Publishers, Chicago, p 1–29

Eward R D 1978 Cauterization of stages I and II endometriosis and the resulting pregnancy rate. In: Phillips J (ed) Endoscopy in gynecology, American Association of Gynecological Laparoscopists, Downey, California, p 276–278

Feste J 1984 Laser laparoscopy. Fertility and Sterility 41:745 (abstract)

Frangenheim H 1972 Laparoscopy and culdoscopy in gynaecology, Butterworths, London, p 35–40

Fraser H M 1983 Effect of treatment for one year with a luteinizing hormone-releasing hormone agonist on ovarian thyroidal and adrenal function and menstruation in the stimptailed monkey (Macaca arctoides) Endocrinology 112:245–253

Fraser I, Allen J K 1979 Danazol and cholesterol metabolism. Lancet 1:931

Fraser I S, Weisberg E 1981 A comprehensive review of injectable contraceptives with special emphasis on depo medroxyprogesterone acetate. Medical Journal of Australia. January, 1981 special suppl

Garcia C D, David S S 1977 Pelvic endometriosis: infertility and pelvic pain. American Journal of Obstetrics and Gynecology 129:740–747

Gjönnaess H 1984 Polycystic ovarian syndrome treated by ovarian electrocautery through the laparoscope. Fertility and Sterility 41:20–25

Gomel V 1980 The impact of microsurgery on gynecology. Clinical Obstetrics and Gynecology 23:1301–1310

Grant A 1963 An evaluation of the conservative treatment of endometriosis. Australian and New Zealand Journal of Obstetrics and Gynaecology 3:162–167

Greenblatt R B, Dmowski L P, Mahesh U, Scholer H F C 1971 Clinical studies with an anti gonadotrophin—danazol. Fertility and Sterility 22:102–113

Greenblatt R B, Tzingounis U 1979 Danazol treatment of endometriosis longterm follow-up. Fertility and Sterility 32:518–520

Grimes D A, Peterson H B 1982 Should dilation and curettage be performed routinely at the time of laparoscopy? Journal of Reproductive Medicine 27:213–216

Hammond C B, Rock J A, Parker R J 1976 Conservative treatment of endometriosis: the effects of limited surgery and hormonal pseudopregnancy. Fertility and Sterility 27:756–766

Hersh L B, McKelvy J F 1979 Enzymes involved in the degrading of thyrotrophin-releasing hormone (THR) and luteinizing hormone-releasing hormone (LHRH) in bovine brain. Brain Research 168:553–564

Jenkin G 1980 Review: the mechanism of action of danazol, a novel steroid derivative. Australian and New Zealand Journal of Obstetrics and Gynaecology 20:113–118

Joel-Cohen S J 1978 The place of the abdominal hysterectomy. Clinics in Obstetrics and Gynecology 5:525–543

Johnston W 1976 Dydrogesterone and endometriosis. British Journal of Obstetrics and Gynaecology 83:77–80

Kable W T, Yussman M A 1981 Fertility after conservative treatment of endometriosis, an analysis of 140 cases. Fertility and Sterility 35:(suppl) 265 (abstract)

Karnaky K J 1948 Use of stilboestrol for endometriosis. Southern Medical Journal 41:1109–1111

Kelly R W, Roberts D K 1983 Experiences with the carbon dioxide laser in gynaecological microsurgery. American Journal of Obstetrics and Gynecology 146:585–588

Keye W R, Matson G A, Dixon J 1983 The rise of argon laser in the treatment of experimental endometriosis. Fertility and Sterility 39:26–27

Khoo S K, Mackay E V, Adam R R 1971 Contraception with a six monthly injection of progesterone. Part III. Effects in the endometrium. Australian and New Zealand Journal of Obstetrics and Gynaecology 11:226–232

Kistner R W 1958 The use of newer progestins in the treatment of endometriosis. American Journal of Obstetrics and Gynecology 75:264–278

Kistner R W 1975 Management of endometriosis in the infertile patient. Fertility and Sterility 26:1151–1161

Koch Y, Baram T, Chobsieng P, Fridkin M 1974 Enzymatic degradation of luteinizing hormone-releasing hormone (LHRH) by hypothalamic tissue. Biochemical and Biophysical Research Communications 61:95–103

Lemay A, Quesnel G 1982 Potential new treatment for endometriosis: reversible inhibition of pituitary ovarian function by chronic intranasal administration of luteinizing hormone (LHRH) agonist. Fertility and Sterility 38:376–379

Lemay A, Faure N, Labrie I, Falekas A 1983 Gonadotrophins and corpus luteum responses to two successive intranasal doses of LHRH agonist at different days after the mid cycle LHRH surge. Fertility and Sterility 39:661–667

Lemay A, Maheux R, Faure N, Jean C, Fazekas A T A 1984 Reversible hypogonadism induced by a luteinizing hormone-releasing hormone (LHRH) agonist (Buserelin) as a new therapeutic approach for endometriosis. Fertility and Sterility 41:863–871

Luciano A A, Houser K S, Chapler F K, Davis W A, Wallace R B 1983 Effects of danazol on plasma lipos and lipoprotein levels in healthy women and in women with endometriosis. American Journal of Obstetrics and Gynecology 145:422–426

McArthur J W, Ulfelder H 1965 The effect of pregnancy in endometriosis. Obstetrical and Gynaecological Survey 20:709–733

McLaughlin D S 1984 Evaluation of adhesion formation by early second laparoscopy following microlaser ovarian wedge resection. Fertility and Sterility 41:465 (abstract)

Meigs J V 1938 Endometriosis, a possible etiological factor. Surgery, Gynaecology and Obstetrics 67:253 (editorial)

Meigs J V 1949 Panel discussion on endometriosis. Journal of American Medical Association 139:975–976

Meldrum D R, Chang R J, Lu J, Vale W, Rivier J, Judd H L 1982 Medical oophrectomy using a long acting GnRH agonist—a possible new approach to the treatment of endometriosis. Journal of Clinical Endocrinology and Metabolism 54:1081–1083

Meldrum D R, Pardridge W M, Kadow W G, Rivier J, Vale W, Judd H L 1983 Hormonal effects of danazol and medical oophorectomy in endometriosis. Obstetrics and Gynaecology 62:480–485

Mettler L, Semm K 1979 Clinical and biochemical experiences with danazol in the treatment of endometriosis in cases with female infertility. Postgraduate Medical Journal 55:(suppl) 22–32

Mildwisky A, Besch N F, Besch P K, Kaufman R 1983 Evidence of a possible direct action of danazol in the human ovary. Acta Obstetrica et Gynecologica Scandinavica 62:187–190

Millar D R 1978 The use of laparoscopy in gynaecology. Clinics in Obstetrics and Gynaecology 5:571–590

Moghissi K S, Boyce C R 1976 Management of endometriosis with oral medroxyprogesterone acetate. Obstetrics and Gynaecology 47:265–267

Moghissi K S, Wallach E 1983 Unexplained infertility. Fertility and Sterility 39:5–21

Moore E E, Harger J H, Rock J A, Archer D F 1981 Management of pelvic endometriosis with low dose danazol. Fertility and Sterility 36:15–19

Morrison J C, Martin D C, Blair R H et al 1980 The use of medroxyprogesterone acetate for relief of symptoms. American Journal of Obstetrics and Gynecology 138:99–104

Noble A D, Letchworth A T 1980 Treatment of endometriosis: a study of medical management. British Journal of Obstetrics and Gynaecology 87:726–728

Nordenskjold F, Ahlgren M 1983 Laparoscopy in female infertility. Acta Obstetrica et Gynecologica Scandinavica 62:609–615

Paterson M E C, Jordan J A, Logan-Edwards R 1978 A survey of 100 patients who had laparoscopic ventrosuspensions. British Journal of Obstetrics and Gynaecology 85:468–471

Polan M, de Cherney A 1980 Presacral neurectomy for pelvic pain in infertility. Fertility and Sterility 321:557–560

Portuondo J A, Navarra E, Benito J A, Obregon M J 1982 Indications for and limitations of laparoscopic ovarian biopsy. Journal of Reproductive Medicine 27:67–72

Portuondo J A, Echanojauregui A D, Herran C, Alijarte I 1983 Early conception in patients with untreated mild endometriosis. Fertility and Sterility 39:22–25

Pratt J H, Williams T J 1980 Indications for complete pelvic operations and more radical procedures in the treatment of severe or extensive endometriosis. Clinical Obstetrics and Gynecology 23:937–950

Puleo J G, Hammond C B 1983 Conservative treatment of endometriosis externa: the effects of danazol therapy. Fertility and Sterility 40:164–169

Pusey J, Taylor P, Leader A, Pattison H A 1984 Outcome and effects in women with infertility following removal of an ectopic pregnancy. American Journal of Obstetrics and Gynecology 148:524–527

Puolakka J, Kauppila A, Ronnberg L 1980 Results in the operative treatment of endometriosis. Acta Obstetrica et Gynecologica Scandinavica 59:429–431

Rantala M L, Kahanpaa K V, Koskimies A, Widholm O 1983 Fertility prognosis after surgical treatment of pelvic endometrioisis. Acta Obstetrica et Gynecologica Scandinavica 62:11–14

Ratsula, K, Haukkamaa M, Wickmann K, Kuukkainen T 1983 Vaginal contraception with gossypol, a clinical study. Contraception 27:571–576

Raynaud J P, Ojasoo T 1983 Promegestone: a new progestin. Journal de Gynecologie Obstetric et Biologie de la Reproduction 12:697–710

Richards B 1978 Hysterectomy: from women to women. American Journal of Obstetrics and Gynecology 131:446–449

Rock J A, Guzick D S, Sengos G, Schweditsch M, Sapp K C, Jones H W 1981 The conservative surgical treatment of endometriosis: evaluation of pregnancy success with respect to the extent of disease as categorized using contemporary classification symptoms. Fertility and Sterility 30:545–548

Rosenfield A G 1974 Injectable long acting progestogen contraception, a neglected modality. American Journal of Obstetrics and Gynecology 120:537–548

Rossman F, D'Ablaing G, Marks R P 1983 Pregnancy complicated by ruptured endometrioma. Obstetrics and Gynaecology 62:519–521

Sadigh H, Naples J D Jr, Batt R E 1977 Conservative surgery for endometriosis in the infertile couple. Obstetrics and Gynaecology 49:562–566

Schenken R S, Malinak L R 1978 Reoperation after initial treatment of endometriosis with conservative surgery. American Journal of Obstetrics and Gynecology 131:416–424

Schenken R S, Malinak L R 1982 Conservative surgery versus expectant management for the infertile patient with mild endometriosis. Fertility and Sterility 37:183–196

Schiff I, Tulchinsky D, Cramer D, Ryan K J 1980 Oral progesterone in treatment of post menopausal symptoms. Journal of the American Medical Association 244:1443–1445

Schmidt-Gollwitzer M, Hardt W, Schmidt-Gollwitzer K, Von dor Ohe M, Nevinny-Stickel J 1981 Influence of the LHRH analogue Buserelin on cyclic ovarian function and on endometrium. A new approach to fertility control. Contraception 23:187–195

Semm K 1975 Atlas of gynecological laparoscopy and hysteroscopy. W B Saunders and Co, Philadelphia, p 232–235

Semm K, Mettler L 1980 Technical progress in pelvic surgery via operative laparoscopy. American Journal of Obstetrics and Gynecology 138:121–127

Shaw R W, Fraser H M 1984 Intranasal treatment with luteinizing hormone releasing hormone agonist in women with endometriosis. Journal of Steroid Biochemistry 20:1403

Shaw R W, Fraser K M, Boyle H 1983 Intranasal treatment with luteinizing hormone releasing hormone agonist in women with endometriosis. British Medical Journal 287:1667–1669

Shaw R W, Kerr-Wilson R H J, Fraser H M, McNeilly A S, Howie P W, Sandow J 1985 Effect of an intranasal LHRH agonist on gonadotrophins and hot flushes in post-menopausal women. Maturitas 7:161–167

Sherman D, Langer R, Sadovsky G, Bukovsky I, Caspi E 1982 Improved fertility following ectopic pregnancy. Fertility and Sterility 37:497–502

Siebel M M, Berger M J, Weinstein F G, Taylor M L 1982 The effectiveness of danazol on subsequent fertility in minimal endometriosis. Fertility and Sterility 38:534–537

Sloan D 1978 The emotional and psychosexual aspects of hysterectomy. American Journal of Obstetrics and Gynecology 131:598–605

Smith T 1978 The surgical treatment of endometriosis. Clinics in Obstetrics and Gynecology 5:557–570

Steptoe P C 1967 Laparoscopic surgical technique. In: Laparoscopy in gynaecology, Livingstone, London, p 72–80

Sulewski J M, Curcio F D, Bronitsky, Stenger V G 1980 The treatment of endometriosis at laparoscopy for infertility. American Journal of Obstetrics and Gynecology 138:128–132

Surrey M W, Breedman S 1982 Second look laparoscopy after reconstructive pelvic surgery for infertility. Journal of Reproductive Medicine 27:651–660

Sutton C 1974 Limitation of laparoscopic ovarian biopsy. Journal of Obstetrics and Gynaecology of the British Commonwealth 81:317–320

Sutton C 1984 Personal communication

Toppozada M, Parman C, Fotherby K 1978 Effects of injectable contraceptives

Endometriosis

Depo-Provera and norethisterone oenanthate on pituitary gonadotrophic response to LHRH. Fertility and Sterility 30: 545–548

van Zyl J A, Muller M A, van Niekerk W A 1980 Danazol in the treatment of endometriosis externa. South African Medical Journal 58: 591–598

Venter B 1980 Endometriosis. South African Medical Journal 57: 895–899

Wahl P, Walden C, Knopp R et al 1983 The effects of oestrogen/progestin potency in lipid/lipoprotein cholesterols. New England Journal of Medicine 308: 862–867

Ward G 1979 Dosage aspects of danazol therapy in the treatment of endometriosis. Postgraduate Medical Journal 55: (Suppl 5) 7–9

Wheeler J A, Malinak L R 1981 Postoperative danazol therapy in infertility patients with severe endometriosis. Fertility and Sterility 38: 543–547

Wheeler J A, Malinak L R 1983 Recurrent endometriosis, incidence, management and prognosis. American Journal of Obstetrics and Gynecology 146: 247–250

Wheeler J A, Johnston B M, Malinak L R 1983 The relationship of endometriosis to spontaneous abortion. Fertility and Sterility 39: 656–666

Williams T A, Ederson J, Ross R J 1978 A radio immunoassay for danazol. Steroids 31: 205–217

Winston R M L 1978 The future of microsurgery in infertility. Clinics in Obstetrics and Gynecology 5: 607–622

7

Hindsight

It was hoped that this study would answer some of the puzzles about endometriosis, enlighten and illuminate the 'grey areas', and leave a tidy current review of endometriosis.

Some salient features that came out of this study were that no ethnic group seems to be particularly vulnerable, or particularly invulnerable to endometriosis and about one in 10 women from the menarche to the menopause in most communities can be expected to have endometriosis, except for those who have a mother, sister, or daughter with the disease, in which case the incidence may double to one in five. More work is needed on the possible genetic inheritance factors. One in 20 sufferers will be teenagers for whom the management includes long-term suppression of menses as well as conservative surgery. Progestogens offer the most satisfactory method of producing long periods of amenorrhoea in this age group in whom coincidental disease processes were unusually common: 8% had cervical dysplasia, a pathological phenomenon in sexually active youngsters noted world-wide in recent times. The menopause, even without oestrogen replacement therapy, does not offer a guaranteed escape from endometriosis which needs to be considered in the differential diagnosis of gynaecological symptoms and signs for up to several years after the menopause.

Some 80% of patients in the Brisbane series had taken oral contraceptive pills, 54% were parous and many had lactated so prior pill use, pregnancy and lactation do not necessarily protect against the development of endometriosis. There was no particular difference in the incidence of recorded spontaneous abortions before and after treatment of endometriosis in the Brisbane series, but ectopic pregnancy was more than twice as common after reparative and reconstructive surgery, presumably due to further interference with tubal physiology as a result of surgery. Recurrent disease repeatedly occurred after successful pregnancy in this series confirming that pregnancy does not protect against endometriosis although it may delay the onset.

Adenomyosis and fibroids were not found in association with endometriosis as commonly as was expected but the coincident association with polycystic ovary disease, present in about one in 12 patients in the author's practice was quite dramatic, especially as about one-half of the patients with polycystic ovary disease had endometriosis, and one-third of the patients with endometriosis had polycystic ovary disease. This relationship needs further-clarification.

Laparoscopy has had a most dramatic effect on both the earlier diagnosis, and treatment at an earlier stage of the disease and approximately one in four patients having a laparoscopic examination may be expected to show endometriosis. Clinical examination has been demonstrated to be unreliable in establishing an accurate diagnosis in both abdominal pain and infertile patients with an error rate of 17 to 63% false positive or false negative findings, and therefore laparoscopic examination is mandatory to establish accurate diagnoses in infertility patients and women with pelvic pain.

Tantalizing research has opened up new avenues for further exploration in relation to endometriosis and possible immune dysfunction, and the significance of peritoneal macrophages and complement (C3, C4) has to be further defined. Prostaglandin production and activity and its precise relationship to endometriosis and infertility has to be determined, while the so-called luteinized unruptured follicle syndrome seems, in Australia at least, to be little more than an occasional phenomenon rather than a clearly defined syndrome, and probably has little direct significance in endometriosis. There may be a connection between infertility and the production of endometriosis due to luteal inadequacy and progestin deficiency. The link between genetic factors, and dopamine exhaustion factors and CNS control cells in FSH/LH production in both polycystic ovary disease and endometriosis needs to be further pursued and evaluated in depth.

The earliest demonstrated stage in the life history of endometriosis—stage 0 disease or occult endometriosis—has been recorded for the first time and a suggested staging system related to the extent of disease and degree of organ destruction and loss of function has been demonstrated. As yet there is no uniformly acceptable classification or staging system available so it is even more difficult to compare results of treatment modalities between centres, given the variability in surgical standards already existing.

Endometriosis arising in post-tubal electrocautery fistulae needs to be distinguished from endosalpingiosis, an entirely different disease. Malignancy and endometriosis rarely coexisted in the Brisbane series although the only death occurred due to carcinoma arising in a conserved fallopian tube following hysterectomy and unilateral adnexectomy for stage II disease 2 years previously. Clinically, 22% of patients in the Brisbane series had no symptoms and 13% had no signs. The so-called classical picture of endometriosis occurred in only 4% of patients casting doubts on its significance. Endometriosis is a protean, not a precise disease.

Treatment, individualized according to the patient's wishes, her age, parity, fertility needs and so forth should be primarily surgical with adjunctive medical therapy. Surgery ranges from conservative at initial laparoscopy for minor disease, through microsurgical/Laser reparative and reconstructive surgery at laparotomy for destructive disease, to radical ablative surgery for extensive disease, or in those who wish it. It is possible that for disease that is classified as stage II or worse, unilateral adnexal disease is better treated by resection rather than repair for improved fertility results. Laser surgery will produce better results than orthodox surgery at all stages of endometriosis and Laser laparoscopy looks to be an exciting prospect for the future. Successful pregnancy is not the only parameter of cure since not every endometriosis victim is in a position to, or wishes to, conceive. Medical treatment prior to conception, or for long-term control, is best maintained using progestins. Danazol does more harm than good and 'medical oophorectomy' using gonadotrophin releasing hormone agonists needs further research. Progestins are effective in those having radical surgery to control post-castration symptoms or to prevent recurrent disease when ovarian tissue is preserved at hysterectomy.

The role of appendicectomy in endometriosis surgery has been discussed. In the Brisbane series the appendix was involved as often as the bowel and therefore appendicectomy was commonly performed. However, in surgery for infertility the appendix should only be removed when it is the site of obvious disease, otherwise fertility may be further compromised by unwitting faecal contamination at appendicectomy.

Presacral neurectomy, while advocated by many endometriosis surgeons elsewhere, has never been used in the Brisbane series without, it is believed, having compromised the patients' well-being.

Endometriosis

There remain many unanswered questions about endometriosis. It seems that about 60% of patients with the disease will reproduce successfully if they have the earlier stages of the disease, and as few as 30% with severe disease will be successful. Despite reproduction, the disease will probably recur in at least 40% of patients and repeated surgical attacks seem to offer reasonable hopes of success in terms of pregnancy outcome for about 30–40% of patients but there is still no single operation and no single drug that is 100% effective for all patients with all stages of endometriosis.

Some of the myths of endometriosis need to be buried. It is not only a disease of private patients in affluent societies; it occurs most often before the age of 30 years and can exist after the menopause; it is not confined to thin, tense, over-achievers attempting initial conception late in life as my plump 34-year-old gravida 10 patient can testify; it is not prevented by contraceptive pills, pregnancy or lactation; and it is becoming more common because women in general have greater expectations of gynaecological good health; clinicians are more aware of the clues that may lead to a diagnosis of endometriosis; and laparoscopy is more readily available universally for the early diagnosis and treatment of the disease at an earlier stage.

The author knows of no women who following the surgical diagnosis of endometriosis has had a proven spontaneous remission prior to the menopause without the influence of pregnancy, surgery, or medical treatment. Therefore endometriosis remains a ubiquitous, enigmatic, malevolent and relentless disease process. Sir William Osler in 1903 wrote 'In the practice of medicine the education of the heart must keep pace with the education of the mind.' Alexis Carrel (1873–1944) said 'a few observations and much reasoning leads to error; many observations and a little reasoning, to truth'. It is hoped that this study reinforces both of these statements.

REFERENCES

Carrel 1968 Quoted in: Strauss M B (ed) Familiar medical quotations. Little Brown, Boston, p 336
Osler W 1903 On the educational value of the Medical Society. Aequanimitas, 3rd ed. McGraw Hill, New York, p 337

INDEX

Abortion and endometriosis, 16
  prostaglandin levels, 33
Acosta classification, 57
Acute abdomen as sign, 77–78
Adenomyomas, disseminated,
  abdominal and pelvic, 50
Adenomyosis and endometriosis, 17,
  146
  coexistent, 50
  in non-human primates, 21–22
Adhesions in endometriosis, 38–39
Adnexal signs, 78
Adolescent patient, 8–11
  coincidental pathology, 9–11
  emotional needs, 10
  management factors, 10–11
Aetiology and pathogenesis, 24–43
  definition, 25
  hypothalamo-pituitary-ovarian axis
    factors, 33–38
  immunological considerations, 29–31
  luteinized unruptured follicle
    syndrome, 26–29
    see also Luteinized unruptured
    follicle syndrome
  mechanical implantation factors, 38–
    39
  ovarian morphology and function,
    26–29
  prostaglandin, role, 32–33
  steroid receptors, 39–40
Age incidence, 8–13
American Fertility Society
  classification, 59–60
  modification, 60–63
Amniocentesis needle tracks, 38
Anaesthesia in laparoscopy, 81
Androgen activity generated by
  progestogens, 116
Appendicectomy, 147
  in endometriosis with infertility, 51–
    52
Autoimmune response, 30–31

Blackledge syndrome and
  endometriosis, 9
Bladder in endometriosis, 53
Bowel involvement in endometriosis, 51
Brisbane series, 2–4
  Danazol results, 124
  early hormone treatment, 5
  population factors, 3–4
  practice arrangements, 3
  progestogen therapy, 114
  questions asked, 6
  records and record analysis, 4–6
    computer system, 5
Bromocriptine in galactorrhoea and
  infertility, 33
Buserelin in endometriosis, 132–136
  circulating oestradiol levels, 132–133
  endometriosis symptoms, 134–135
  endometriotic deposit changes, 135–
    136
  uterine bleeding patterns, 133

Caesarean section scars, 38
Carbon dioxide laser wedge technique,
  37–38, 94–96
Carcinoid tumour, 51
Catamenial pneumothorax, 52
Cervical intra-epithelial neoplasia and
  endometriosis, 9, 10
Classification of endometriosis, 57–64
  see also Staging
Clear cell cancer, 55
Clinical features
  signs, 75–78
  symptoms, 68–75
Clomiphene citrate in PCOD, 37
Complement system in endometriosis,
  31, 146
  C3 and C4 concentrations, 31
Computer system, 5
Contraception
  hormonal, endometriosis and, 13
  oral, effects, 145–146

Index

Contraception (cont.)
  pharmacology, 114–117
    atherogenicity, 117–118
    combination, and
      pseudopregnancy, 118
    didrogesterone, 122–123
    medroxyprogesterone acetate, 120–
      122
    northisterone (and acetate), 116,
      118, 121, 122
    progestogens alone, 119–120
  preparations in therapy, 113–114
Cure rate, 104–105

Danazol (Danocrine/Danol) in
    pseudomenopause in
    endometriosis therapy, 123–129,
    147
  Brisbane series, 124
  comparative study, 125
  comparison with GnRH agonist, 127–
    129
  fertility outcome, 125
  half-life, 125
  long-term usage, 124–125
  recurrence, 126
  side effects, 126–127
  variability of laboratory results, 123
Definition, 25
Depo-Provera in endometriosis, 120–
    122
Deposits, endometriotic changes during
    LHRH agonist treatment, 135
Diagnosis, 78–83
  differential, 83
  laparoscopy, 81–82
  nuclear magnetic resonance imaging,
    80–81
  at other operations, 82–83
  peritoneal flushing and cytology, 79
  surgery, Brisbane, 78
    at other operations, 82–83
  ultrasound, 80
Didrogesterone in endometriosis, 122–
    123
Diethylstilboestrol exposure, 18–19
Differential diagnosis, 83
Dilatation and curettage (D & C) with
    laparoscopy, 89
Dysmenorrhoea as symptom, 68–70
Dyspareunia as symptom, 71

Ectopic pregnancies, laparotomy,
    microsurgery, 93, 94

Electrocautery, post-tubal, 147
Endometrioid cancer, 54–55, 56, 57
Endometriomata, removal, 102–103
Endometriosis, treatment, 85–143
  see also Treatment
Endometriotic polyposis, 56
Endocervicosis, 46–47
Endosalpingosis, 46–50
  histogenesis, 46
  incidence, 48
  oviduct endometriosis, differential
    diagnosis, 47–48
  psammoma bodies, 46
  serous tumours and, 46
Enovid therapy, 113
Enzyme deficiencies in polycystic ovary
    disease, 35–36
Epidemiology, 7–23
  age incidence, 8–13
  coincidental disease, 17–18
  exploratory surgery, incidence of
    endometriosis, 19–20
  heritable factors, 14
  immunosuppressive drug therapy, 13–
    14
  in the male, 20
  in non-human primates, 20–22
  parity, 15–17
  previous pelvic surgery, 15
  vaginal adenosis, 18
Episiotomy scars, 38
Ethnic factors, 7–8, 145
Exploratory surgery, incidence of
    endometriosis, 19–20

Fibroids
  endometriosis and, 17–18, 146
  polycystic ovary disease and, 18
Follicle(s), in polycystic ovary disease,
    35–36
  stimulating hormone levels, 36
    /LH link with other factors, 146
    Gossypol and, 138

Galactorrhoea-endometriosis, 33, 74–75
Genital tract
  congenital anomalies, 18
  epithelial dysplasia, 19
Gestrinone in treatment, 137
Glucuronide levels, 34
Gonadotrophin releasing hormone,
    (GnRH)
  agonist in endometriosis, 127–129
    compared with Danazol, 127–129
  stimulation, 36

Gossypol in treatment, 137–138
Guildford, England, endometriosis
  incidence in, 1

Heart transplant, endometriosis and, 29
Heritable factors in endometriosis, 14
Historical factors, 24–25
Hormone treatment, early, Brisbane, 5
Hydroxyprogesterone therapy, 113
Hyperprolactinaemic galactorrhoea and
  endometriosis, 33
  bromocriptine, 33
Hypothalamo-pituitary-ovarian axis
  factors, 33–38
Hysterectomy
  complications, 111
  emotional aspects, 97–100
  endometriosis and, 12
    diagnosis, 82–83
  indications, 100–103
  results, 105–106

Immunoglobulins, 30
Immunological considerations, 29–31,
  146
Immunosuppressive drug therapy prior
  to diagnosis, 13–14
Infertility
  appendicectomy and, 51–52
  aspects of treatment, 85–86
  endometriosis and, 15–17
  laparoscopy, 87–92
    see also Laparoscopy
  laparotomy, 92–96
    see also Laparotomy
  primary surgery
    with fertility preservation, 106–
    107
      pregnancy outcome, 106–107
      relation to recurrence, 108–110
    without fertility preservation, 106
  as symptom, 71–72
  use of Danazol, 125
Intestinal endometriosis, 50–52

6-Keto-prostaglandin F levels in
  endometriosis, 32
Kistner classification, 58–59

Laparoscopy, 146
  in adolescence, 6
  complications, 110

in diagnosis, 2, 81–82
incidence, shown, 82
in treatment, 87–92
  abdominal stab wounds, 90
  additional procedures, 89–90
  benefits, 91–92
  cost factors, 91
  dilatation and curettage (D&C)
    with, 89
  instruments, 89
  technique, 88–89
Laparotomy as diagnostic procedure,
  82–83, 92–96
  complications, 111
  in infertility, 92–96
    factors to produce good
      pregnancy rates, 92–93
    lasers, 94–96
    microsurgery, 93–94
Laser techniques in surgery, 37–38, 94–
  96, 147
Leiomyomata and endometriosis, 17
Lipoproteins, LDL, HDL, VLDL,
  atherogenicity of sex steroids,
  117–118
Location of endometriosis, 45
Luteal inadequacy and endometriosis,
  34
Luteinized unruptured follicle (LUF),
  26–29
  in aetiology of endometriosis, 26–27
  incidence, 27–28
    ultrasound diagnosis, 28
  role of ovarian steroids, 27, 28
  steroid hormone assay, 27
  syndrome, 18
Luteinizing hormone levels in
  endometriosis, 34, 35, 36
  sleep pattern, 36
  surges, 36
Luteinizing hormone releasing hormone
  agonist in endometriosis, 129–
  132
  Buserelin, 132–136
    see also Buserelin
  effect on gonadotrophin secretion,
    130–132
  in postmenopause, 130
  in premenopause, 130

Macrophages, pelvic and peritoneal,
  29–30
Male, endometriosis in, 20

Malignant tumours in endometriosis, 54–57
transformation, 57
Medical oophorectomy
changes in endometriotic deposits, 135–136
circulating oestradiol levels, 132–133
endometriosis symptoms, 134–135
with GnRH agonist, 127–129, 147
compared with Danazol, 127–129
with LNRH agonist, 129–132
Medroxyprogesterone
acetate as contraceptive, effect on endometriosis, 120–122
in adolescent age group, 11
Menarche, average age and endometriosis, 12–13
Menopause, *see* Pseudomenopause
Menorrhagia as symptom, 73
Menstrual cycle, altered, as symptom, 73–74
Microscopic appearance, 45–46
Multiparity, 50
Muscinous cancer, 55

Needle aspiration of cysts, 90–91
Nodularity as sign, 76
Northisterone (and acetate) in endometriosis treatment, 116, 118, 121, 122
Nuclear magnetic resonance imaging in diagnosis, 80–81

Obesity, PCOD, endometriosis and, 37
Oestradiol
circulating levels during LHRH agonist treatment, 132–133
implants in monkeys, 22
Oestriol-16-gluceronide levels, 34
Oestrogen
atherogenicity, 117
effect on progesterone receptor synthesis, 114–116
effect on progestogenic agents, 116
receptors, 40
Oligomenorrhoea, 74
Oophorectomy, bilateral, in treatment, 97
see also Medical oophorectomy
Ovarian
biopsy, 90
cancer, 55
morphology and function, 26–29

Pain
in dysmenorrhoea, as symptom, 68–70
pelvic, as symptom, 72
Parity and endometriosis, 15–17
Pathogenesis, 24–43
see also Aetiology and pathogenesis
Pathology, 44–57
gross, 44–50
malignant tumours, 54–57
microscopic appearance, 45–46
non-carcinomatous tumour, 56–57
in other organs, 50–54
Pelvic
inflammatory disease in endometriosis, 9, 17, 72–73
pain as symptom, 72–73
surgery, endometriosis development and, 15
Peritoneal flushing and cytology in diagnosis, 79
Pneumothorax, catamenial, 52
Polycystic ovary disease and endometriosis, 9, 11, 17, 34–38
enzyme deficiencies, 35–36
fibroids and, 18
hormonal inter-relationships, 36–37
hypothalamic defect, 37
management, 37–38
obesity, 37
Polypoid endometriosis, 56
Population factors, Brisbane, 3–4
Postmenopause, 11–12
coincidental pathology, 12
oestrogen replacement therapy, 11–12
Post-tubal electrocautery, 147
Pouch of Douglas, tenderness as sign, 76
Pregnancy
after primary surgery, 106–107
drug therapy, 110
relationship to subsequent recurrent disease, 108–110
ectopic, endometriosis diagnosis and, 16–17
outcome, before endometriosis diagnosis, 16
see also Pseudopregnancy
Pregnanediol-3 levels, 34
Premenstrual spotting as symptom, 75
Presacral neurectomy, 102, 147
Primates, non-human, endometriosis in, 20–22
Progesterone
implants in monkeys, 22
receptor synthesis, influence of steroids, 114–116

Progestin
  receptors, 40
  therapy, 113
Progestogens, 147
  alone, 119–120
  in combination oral contraceptives,
    118–119
  oestrogenic effect, 116–117
  pharmacology, 114–117
    derivation, 114, 115
    effect of oestrogen, 114
    potency of compounds, 114
    receptor binding, 114
  therapy, 104
Promegestone in treatment, 138
Prostaglandin
  levels, 74
    raised, 32–33
  role in endometriosis, 32–33
  spontaneous abortion and, 33
Psammoma bodies, 46
Pseudomenopause therapy, Danazol,
  123–129
  see also Danazol (Danocrine/Danol)
Pseudopregnancy therapy, 112–123
  atherogenicity of sex steroids, 117–
    118
  combination oral contraceptives, 118–
    119
  didrogesterone, 122–123
  Enovid, 113
  medroxyprogesterone acetate, 120–
    122
  northisterone (and acetate), 116, 118,
    121, 122
  oral contraceptives, 113–114
  with progestogens alone, 119–120
  progestogen pharmacology, 114–117

Rectovaginal septum, tenderness as
  sign, 76–77
Recurrence, 86–87
  after Danazol, 126
  after surgery, 107–108
  relationship to pregnancy, 108–110
  2nd, 3rd and 4th operations, 107–108
Re-operation, 96

Salpingo-oophorectomy, bilateral,
  results, 106
Sarcomas, endometrial, 55
Serous tumours, 46, 55
Signs, 75–78
  no signs, 75–76

Spotting, premenstrual, as symptom, 75
Staging, 57–64, 146–147
  Acosta, 57–58
  American Fertility Society, 59–60
    modification, 60–63
  Brisbane series, 63–64
  clustering techniques, 62
  Kistner, 58–59
Steroid(s)
  classification, 40
  receptors in endometriosis, 39–40
  sex, atherogenicity, 117–118
Surgery in diagnosis, 78–79, 82
  in PCOD, 37
  in treatment, 87–111, 148
    complications, 110–111
    conservative, 87–96
      laparoscopy, 87–92
      see also Laparoscopy
      laparotomy, 92–96
      see also Laparotomy
    radical, 97–103
    re-operation, 96
    results, 103–111
      cure rate, 104
      fertility not preserved, 106
      pregnancy outcome, 106–107
      recurrence, 107–108
    see also Exploratory, Pelvic
Symptoms, 68–75
  clusters, 69
  during and after treatment with
    LHRH agonist, 134–135
  no symptoms, 71

Tenderness in pouch of Douglas and
  rectovaginal septum as sign, 76–
  77
Thoracic endometriosis, 52
Thromboxane B2 levels in
  endometriosis, 32
Treatment, 85–143
  flow chart for management, 88
  in infertility, 85–86
  medical, 112–129
    Gestrinone, 137
    Gossypol, 137–138
    oophorectomy, 129–136
    see also Medical oophorectomy
    Promegestone, 138
    pseudomenopause therapy, 123–
    129
    Danazol, 123–129

Index

Treatment (cont.)
  pseudopregnancy, 112–123
    atherogenicity of sex steroids, 117–118
    combination oral contraceptives, 118
    didrogesterone, 122–123
    medroxyprogestone acetate, 120–122
    northisterone (and acetate), 116, 118, 121, 122
    progestogens alone, 119–120
    progestogen pharmacology, 114–117
  recurrence, 86–87
  surgery, 87–111
    see also Surgery; and specific techniques

Ultrasound in diagnosis, 80
  in luteinized unruptured follicle diagnosis, 28
Ureteric obstruction, 53
Urinary tract endometriosis, 53–54
Uterine
  bleeding patterns during LHRH agonist treatment, 133–134
  retroversion as sign, 77
  scarring, 38
  signs, 76

Vaginal adenosis, 18–19
Ventrosuspension of retroverted uterus, 90

154